Minski's
Handbook of Psychiat
for
Students and Nurses

Minski's
Handbook of Psychiatry
for
Students and Nurses

SEVENTH EDITION

Robert G. Priest
MD FRCP(E) FRCPsych DPM

*Professor of Psychiatry (University of London),
St Mary's Hospital Medical School,
St Mary's Hospital*

Gerald Woolfson
MB MRCP(G) MRCPsych DPM

*Consultant Psychiatrist and Honorary Senior Lecturer,
The Hammersmith Hospital and Royal Postgraduate Medical School;
Consultant Psychiatrist, Springfield and St Charles Hospitals;
Consultant Psychotherapist, HM Prison, Holloway*

WILLIAM HEINEMANN MEDICAL BOOKS LTD
23 BEDFORD SQUARE, LONDON WC1B 3HH

Printing history
First published as *A Practical Handbook of Psychiatry for Students and Nurses*
by Louis Minski   1946
Second edition 1950, reprinted 1953; Third edition 1956;
Fourth edition 1959, reprinted 1959; Fifth edition 1964,
reprinted 1967; Sixth edition 1973; Seventh edition, revised
and reset 1978, reprinted 1980,
reprinted 1983

ISBN 0 433 26205 2

Text set in 11/12 pt VIP Bembo, printed and bound
in Great Britain at The Pitman Press, Bath

Contents

Preface to the Seventh Edition

The reader will find that we have completely rewritten the text of this book and we have taken the opportunity to bring the accounts of clinical practice and treatment up to date.

We have tried to present concepts that are important, and which are sometimes thought of as difficult, in a way that should be readily understandable to a beginner. We hope that the same virtue of simplicity will make the book valuable to the more advanced reader for use in his revision. For both purposes we have aimed to make what we say immediately comprehensible.

Despite the attractively small size of this book we have covered a large number of facts. To do this we have been didactic and we have concentrated on common practical problems rather than linger on areas of confusing controversy.

Within the subject matter of psychiatry there are certainly topics that are difficult for the beginner to grasp – for instance psychotherapeutic techniques. Where it helps to make ideas clearer we have used a direct person-to-person style more usual in speech than in writing. Although this may be provocative we hope it conveys the meaning with a sense of immediacy. Throughout the book we have tried to provide contact with the subject rather than abstract generalities.

ROBERT PRIEST
GERALD WOOLFSON

Acknowledgements

We are grateful to Marilyn and Lynne for support and encouragement, to Ursula and Nicholas for constructive criticism, and to
countless students (nursing, medical, social work and others) for
letting us know when we were talking clearly and when we were
being obscure. We wish to thank Maria, Jack and Dougal for their
useful advice and Jacky for her patient help in the typing of several
drafts.

We would like to thank Dr Paul Raptopoulos, honorary lecturer
in psychiatry at St Mary's Hospital Medical School, for his help in
the preparation of the index, and Dr John Besford for providing the
artwork.

1 Introduction to Psychiatry

Psychiatry is the branch of medicine that deals with abnormalities of the mind. While a **psychologist** is a scientist who studies the workings of the mind in general (including those of the normal human or even of the animal mind) a **psychiatrist** is a *doctor* who treats diseases, disorders or deficiencies of the human mind.

Abnormal function of the mind shows itself in many different ways. Stress may impair or alter some of the functions of the body, to produce **psychosomatic** disease (such as some cases of peptic ulcer, asthma or skin rashes). In mental deficiency or subnormality the patient is handicapped by an intellect or intelligence that is inadequate for the ordinary needs of everyday life. A mental handicap of this sort is likely to be life-long. However, the majority of psychiatric patients have been relatively well adjusted for most of their lives until the time of their breakdown, so they are said to be suffering from a **mental illness**. The illness is not necessarily severe, and often clears up quite soon. Mild illnesses of this sort are very common and are called **neuroses**. Anxiety states and obsessional neuroses are examples.

More severe mental illnesses are called **psychoses**. In a psychosis the patient often suffers from delusions or hallucinations. A **delusion** is a false belief: the patient may believe his food is being poisoned, that he is riddled with disease, or that he is a person of exalted rank (e.g. royalty). A false belief is accepted as evidence of mental illness only if:

(a) It is held in the face of evidence to the contrary. Many of us from time to time are afraid we may have a disease, but we are usually reassured by negative examination and tests.

(b) It cannot be understood as part of the patient's normal background. Beliefs in witchcraft are quite common in some parts of the world, and would not be regarded as delusional there.

1

Whereas delusions are false beliefs, **hallucinations are false perceptions**. The patient sees, hears, smells, feels or tastes things that are not really there. The normal person does this in dreams, but not usually when fully awake. Healthy people may **misidentify** perceptions – as when we mistake the dressing gown hanging behind the door in dim light for a person standing there. This mistaken sensation is known as an **illusion**, and is part of the stock in trade of the conjurer or stage magician. A genuine hallucination arises spontaneously in the patient's mind, in the absence of an external sensory stimulus, as when the child in a delirium sees strange animals crawling over his bedroom wall.

Some mental illness is caused by disease of the brain. This may be temporary (as with the delirium mentioned above) or it may be permanent (as with the senile changes in old age). These are called **organic** mental illnesses, and usually some alteration in the **structure** of the brain can be demonstrated. Most patients coming up to psychiatric clinics do not have organic brain disorders, and in contrast their mental illnesses are called **functional** (since it is merely the function, not the structure of the brain that is affected).

Psychoses

To sum up so far, the psychoses are more severe than the neuroses, and in particular the patient's contact with reality is more disturbed. Someone suffering from a psychosis may have delusions or hallucinations, whereas a patient with a neurosis has symptoms that are closer to the distress that we all experience from time to time (e.g. anxiety and obsessions). We have seen that delirium and senile dementia are organic psychoses. The functional psychoses include **affective psychosis** and **schizophrenia**.

The word **affect** refers to emotion or mood, and in particular that emotion which can range from depression on the one hand to cheerful elation on the other. In **depressive psychosis** (or melancholia) the patient is typically slowed up in his actions, low in spirits, and suffers from unpleasant thoughts or even delusions that he has incurable disease, that he is in hopeless financial trouble, that he is rotten through and through, or that he has committed unforgiveable sins. This contrasts with the patient with **mania** (or **hypomania** if it is not quite so extreme) who is energetic and overactive, elated, and has grandiose beliefs that he possesses vast wealth or that he is an extremely important person (ideas of grandeur). Depressive psychosis and mania (or hypomania) are together known as the affective psychoses. Some patients experience both extremes at different times (**manic–depressive psychosis**).

Schizophrenia is the other important functional psychosis. Here the typical delusions are much stranger and more difficult to understand. Whereas the delusions in depressive psychosis can be seen to be saddening, and those in hypomania to be cheering, the beliefs of the schizophrenic are characteristically odd. For instance, if a schizophrenic patient believes that there are little men inside the central heating radiators, this is not a particularly cheering or saddening belief so much as a peculiar belief. The behaviour of the schizophrenic patient is as bizzarre as some of his delusional beliefs and his emotions do not fit in with the thoughts he expresses. The central feature of the clinical picture is that it is so 'non-understandable'.

Mental illness and personality disorders

As with any other illness, patients with mental illnesses have *symptoms* – distressing disturbances about which the patient will complain. They include phobias, apprehension, suicidal feelings, insomnia, loss of interest, loss of energy, unpleasant delusions and hallucinations. There is another group of psychological disorders in which the diagnosis is based not on symptoms but on *character traits*. These patients are said to suffer from **personality disorders**. As with mental subnormality (or handicap) these disorders are typically life-long but they show themselves in abnormal behaviour.

There are several differences between character traits and symptoms. Character traits are long lasting: symptoms are often of short duration. Symptoms are distressing to the patient: character traits need not be. We all have character traits: at any given time not all of us have symptoms. These differences mean that it is much more difficult to be sure of a diagnosis of personality disorder than it is of a mental illness. For instance most patients will either definitely have the syptom of palpitations or they will deny having them. Similarly a patient will either hear 'voices' or he will not. But take a character trait such as conscientiousness. We all have varying degrees of conscientiousness. Some of our acquaintances may be extremely conscientious. Others may be conspicuously casual in matters of conscience. It is difficult to decide where the cut-off point should come between normal and abnormal. Who is to say when someone is so crippled by agonies of conscience that he should be regarded as suffering from a pathological state? The decision is clearly subjective and probably is influenced a lot by how conscientious is the observer himself.

In practice, the decision to regard someone as a patient depends not only on the severity of the deviation from average behaviour, but also on such factors as the amount of disability suffered, whether the affected person regards **himself** as needing treatment, whether others suffer as a result of his disorder, and whether the suffering (to the patient or to others) is out of proportion to the circumstances that precipitated it.

Psychopathic personality

Since there are as many character traits as you care to think of, and since each may reach pathological extremes, the term 'personality disorder' includes a large number of varying conditions. One of the most important is known either as **psychopathic personality** or as **sociopathic personality**.

The typical psychopath shows four important characteristics:

1 persistent antisocial behaviour
2 impulsiveness
3 lack of guilt
4 inability to form stable interpersonal relationships based on mutual trust and affection ('lovelessness') (see pp. 84–85).

Such a person may commit a senselessly violent crime, and is as likely to end up in jail as with a psychiatrist. After impulsively committing his antisocial act he will be found to be lacking in remorse or self-reproach. A detailed examination of his life history will show, too, that he never makes true friends, and that he exploits others rather than trusts them. In fact, it is often the case that a diagnosis can only be made by reviewing the individual's life history and cataloguing the repeated episodes of antisocial behaviour.

Another characteristic feature is the poor response to treatment of any kind (see Chs. 17–19). It will be seen that it is often very difficult to fit personality disorders into a diagnostic category.

Personality disorders in medical practice

Patients who are labelled by doctors as 'personality disorders' or even 'psychopaths' have very frequently presented in the first instance with a problem concerning either **sex** or **drugs**. That is to say, although there is no absolute reason why someone with a minority sexual practice (e.g. homosexuality) should not be otherwise well adjusted, a high proportion of those complaining to doctors about such a problem are thought to have disordered personalities of some degree.

This also applies to patients addicted to (physically dependent on) drugs. Patients attending drug dependence clinics with addiction to narcotic drugs (such as heroin) have a particularly high prevalence of disordered personalities, and large numbers of them have been in conflict with the law over other matters before their drug usage started. In developed countries the commonest form of drug dependence is alcoholism. Among alcoholics is found a complete range from those on the one hand with severe personality disorder to those on the other hand who are well within the normal range of character make-up, apart from their vulnerability to alcohol.

The other type of drug problem that is becoming much more prevalent is that of taking overdoses. Some patients taking a single overdose show deviant personalities (others are suffering from a depressive illness or are relatively normal psychologically). Abnormal and antisocial character traits are particularly common among those who take overdoses repeatedly over months or years.

Other personality types

The **obsessional** personality (see pp. 14–15) shows traits of orderliness: he is particularly concerned with punctuality, cleanliness, scrupulousness, and attention to detail. He also often has traits of parsimony (hoarding his money) and stubbornness.

The **hysterical** personality (see pp. 17–18) is attention-seeking, emotional, manipulative and tends to exaggerate and overact. The **schizoid** personality is emotionally cold and uninvolved to the point of being callous. A **depressive** personality has a life-long tendency to pessimism, apathy and lack of energy whereas a **hypomanic** personality has the opposite traits. The **cyclothymic** personality swings (much more than the rest of us) from depressive moods at one time to hypomanic tendencies the next.

One can also describe **anxious, irritable** and **paranoid** personalities. In fact take almost any psychological adjective and you can make up a personality type. You can see that this is not a field where diagnosis is very precise. One of the least satisfactory labels is that of **inadequate personality.** This diagnosis is made when the person concerned does not succeed in life to the level that his intelligence and education would seem to fit him for. To make such a diagnosis calls for so much in the way of judgement and assumptions that it is one of the least reliable of diagnoses in psychiatry.

2 Symptomatology and Mental State

A patient suffering from **anxiety** may be aware of his rapidly pumping heart (palpitations), his excessive perspiration, his shaking hands or of tension pains in the back of his head and neck. All of these are **physical** symptoms of anxiety. The main **mental** symptom of anxiety is *apprehension* – an uncomfortable feeling that something unpleasant might happen. These symptoms may be the only features of the patient's mental illness, in which case they constitute an 'anxiety state'. However, they are very common in all other forms of acute mental illness. So if the patient complains of these symptoms, it is necessary to enquire about possible features of other mental illnesses before coming to the conclusion that 'anxiety state' is the final diagnosis.

If a patient complains of a loss of interest in life, lack of energy, low spirits and feelings of guilt and low self-esteem, we say he is depressed. Once again these symptoms are very common in patients with a variety of diagnoses, so we do not conclude that 'depressive illness' is the diagnosis before going into it further.

How do we assess a patient in order to come to a diagnosis? First of all we take a history. This procedure follows the same outline as in other branches of medicine even though the emphasis may be different. We start by hearing his **presenting complaint** (e.g. palpitations, loss of energy, feelings of persecution) and then ask further questions about it (history of the presenting complaint). To start with this may be an **unstructured interview** in which we ask open-ended questions – e.g. 'Can you tell me some more about that?' – just letting the patient volunteer what comes into his head spontaneously. Later we ask specific or closed questions, to focus down the answers – e.g. 'When did this start?'. We continue by asking about the patient's **past history**, particularly enquiring about any previous treatment for psychiatric disorder (whether from his general practitioner, or in an outpatient clinic, or in a psychiatric unit). Finally we go into the **family history,** not only making enquiries about a family history of mental illness, but also asking about the personalities of the patient's parents and siblings, and the relationship between them, looking for particular causes of conflict.

The next aspect of our assessment is the **mental state examination** (analogous to the physical examination in other branches of medicine). Observation of the patient has naturally been going on while taking the history, so already we can say something about his **appearance** and **behaviour**. Often these features are remarkably normal. Even seriously depressed patients may merely look rather sober or serious: one does not necessarily expect to see weeping or gnashing of teeth, though some patients with depressive psychosis will show **retardation** – a general slowing up of all movements – and some will show **agitation** – purposeless motor activity such as pacing up and down or wringing the hands. The patient may be mute or stuporose. Mutism and stupor may also occur in catatonic schizophrenia, which is also one of the conditions in which the patient may really behave in the way that the lay person thinks of as signifying a 'mental' patient, standing in strange postures or acting in a bizarre manner.

The average psychiatric patient does none of these things, and one may merely note that he has neglected his appearance, or is relatively quiet and unforthcoming on the one hand, or talkative on the other. Analysis of the behaviour of the patient is dealt with further in the section on nursing and management (pp. 171–180).

A great deal of what we learn about the patient comes from his speech. His talk may be retarded in depression. In hypomania it is speeded up, and he changes rapidly from one topic to another in a **flight of ideas**. In schizophrenia the talk is jumbled and may be incomprehensible. This is referred to as disorder of the form of thought, or formal thought disorder, or just as 'thought disorder'. As well as the **flow** and the **form** of expressed thoughts, we also consider thought **content**. In the psychoses the patient suffers from **delusions,** false beliefs inconsistent with the patient's background and the evidence available to him. In paranoid delusions, for instance, the patient believes he is the subject of persecution, people are looking at him, talking about him, and plotting againt him. He may regard a parked car as suspicious, and believe that the occupants are plain clothes detectives following him.

In a **delusional system** one delusion is based on another. Why are detectives following him? The patient with depressive psychosis is likely to attribute the fact to wicked actions that he believes he has committed in the past. The **hypomanic** patient argues that since he is such an important person, yet does not seem to receive the respect that is due to him, it must mean that people have a grudge against him and mean to torment him. The schizophrenic patient, asked to explain why those people are detectives who are following him, may say 'because they are in a yellow car'. This last type of non–understandable belief, not apparently based on anything more fundamental, is known as a **primary delusion**.

Delusions are found only in the psychoses. In the neurotic disorders the patient's thoughts are concerned with his worries, his problems and his symptoms. As part of the mental examination one makes a note of the ideas that are troubling him or with which he is **preoccupied** or excessively **concerned**. These notes are likely to form the largest item in the record of his mental state, and where possible one tries to write down his more important or significant statements word for word. For instance, rather than noting: 'Expresses hostile feelings towards parents' it is preferable to write 'Talking about his family, said "I despise my father and I'm always arguing with my mother" '.

As a rule, when patients are being interviewed, they do not mind notes being made provided the interviewer still continues to pay close attention to what they are saying.

It is usual to write comments on the **affect** of the patient in the mental examination. Your impression of his affect (or mood, or emotional state) comes from observations you have already made under other headings – appearance, behaviour, stream of talk, thought content and so on.

The next step is to see whether he has abnormal perceptions or sensations. Does he have **hallucinations**? You can ask him (if you feel comfortable doing so) if he sees visions, or hears voices that nobody else seems to hear. Hallucinations are conjured up out of nowhere – you could be 'seeing' real looking animals when looking at a plain wall. An **illusion** is a misinterpretation of a real stimulus – you may think that someone is standing behind the bedroom door, but when you put the light on you can see that it is just a dressing gown hanging there. Without illusions there would be no conjurors and of course they are not necessarily a sign of mental illness.

Turning now to the patient's **intellectual functions**, one looks for evidence of mental handicap or subnormality. Can he read and write? If not, and he has had the opportunity to go to school, this suggests a severe intellectual deficit. Otherwise one obtains a general impression of his intelligence by seeing if he uses words correctly, and has a fairly extensive vocabulary. One can look at specific functions, e.g. calculation. Two tests of this are asking the patient to subtract 7 from a hundred, and continue to subtract 7 from each answer in turn (93, 86, 79, 72 etc.), and doubling three, then the answer, and so on (3, 6, 12, 24, 48, 96, 192). On the second test (doubling three) the average person can get into three figures (192 or more) and if the subject cannot reach two figures (12 or more) he is likely to be handicapped.

Since one person may be good at arithmetic but bad at geography, or good at general knowledge but bad at languages, it follows that single tests on their own may be misleading and can give only an approximate idea of the patient's ability. Also, they do not take into account the individual's cultural background. If it is crucial to know his level of intellect more precisely a psychologist administers a battery of tests measuring many different faculties.

If it is suspected that the patient is **dementing**, then special tests (memory, new learning) can be given to detect this (see pp. 66–67). For everyday purposes you can ask the name and address test (see Appendix 1, p. 193).

At this stage it is appropriate to record the patient's orientation in time, place and person.

Finally a note is made about the patient's insight and judgement. 'Insight' is said to be lost in the psychoses, but since the term is used in different ways it is advisable to specify what is meant at the time. For instance, you might write 'Insight impaired, in that he does not seem to realize that he is mentally ill' or 'Accepts that she is depressed but does not realize that she is incontinent'.

Making the diagnosis

As we have seen, anxiety symptoms may occur in most acute mental illnesses, so that we have to **exclude** other diagnoses before giving the patient the label 'anxiety state'. If we find a lot of symptoms of depressive illness, that may be the final diagnosis. Alternatively, a patient who has complained mainly of anxiety and depressive symptoms may be found on mental examination to have hallucinations, delusions and thought disorder of the type found in schizophrenia, in which case this would be the overriding diagnosis.

Finally it should always be remembered that *organic brain disease* can cause any psychiatric symptom, and must therefore always be considered as a possibility. To sum up, neurotic symptoms can be found in psychoses, and any symptoms can be found in organic brain disorder. In making a diagnosis of mental illness, then, the doctor goes down the possible list through progressively more serious conditions, before making up his mind.

A patient with mental illness may suffer from other psychological disorders **as well**. These include mental handicap, personality disorder, psychosomatic disease.

To sum up the case, a psychiatrist may make what is called a 'diagnostic formulation'. One (fictitious) example is as follows:

'A 67 year old widow with a history of peptic ulcer who has an obsessional personality and above average intelligence, presenting ten months after her husband's death in a severe depressive illness with marked phobic features.'

3 Neuroses

Neuroses are less severe than psychoses in the sense that the patient experiences less distortion of reality – for instance, he neither sees visions (hallucinations) nor suffers from mistaken beliefs (delusions) (see pp. 1–2). His experiences are similar to the psychological distress that we all have from time to time.

A neurotic illness takes one of four main forms:

1 Anxiety state
2 Obsessional state
3 Hysteria
4 Depressive illness (neurotic degree)

Anxiety states

In the **phobias** (or phobic anxiety states) the patient is unduly afraid of something specific such as animals or heights. Fears of spiders, or of enclosed spaces, are common in the general population. In some people they are excessive, but it is only when they reach the degree of interfering with ordinary living – for example preventing the patient from getting to work – that they are classified as phobias. A fear of enclosed spaces is known as **claustrophobia**, and a fear of open spaces (often confining the patient to home) is called **agoraphobia**. Phobic anxieties can be treated with anxiety reducing drugs (e.g. diazepam, chlordiazepoxide). Sometimes they respond well to such benzodiazepine tranquillizers combined with a monoamine oxidase inhibitor (MAOI). The action of MAOIs is discussed in the section on antidepressant drugs (pp. 148–149).

Quite a different approach is to treat these disorders with **behaviour therapy**. Here the phobia is seen as a case of **faulty learning**, as if the patient has developed the wrong conditioned responses or reflexes to certain situations. Behaviour therapy is designed to correct the faulty learning, and is discussed more fully as a treatment method elsewhere in this book (p. 159–163).

Apart from the phobias, there are other types of anxiety state. The patient may be excessively concerned about a coming event, such as an examination or a change of job. Anxiety in these circumstances is quite common, so that it is only classified as a neurosis if *the anxiety is excessive in duration or in degree*, in other words quite out of proportion to the real threat.

The emotion of anxiety is different to that of depression. In anxiety the person affected has **an uncomfortable feeling that something unpleasant might happen**. (In depression, the uncomfortable feeling is because something unpleasant has already happened, or is bound to happen.) Other words used to describe this emotion of anxiety are apprehension, dread or fear.

Some patients with anxiety states have this sense of dread, but do not know exactly what it is that they fear. They complain of the emotion of anxiety, and of physical symptoms such as palpitations, sweating or shakiness, without knowing what unpleasant possibility they are scared of facing. This is referred to as **free floating anxiety**.

There is, finally, a most important group of patients who suffer from an anxiety state without even feeling the subjective emotion of anxiety. They merely experience the physical symptoms of anxiety. Among these we have mentioned palpitations, sweating and shakiness; others are dry mouth, diarrhoea and colicky pains, frequency of micturition, difficulty in getting off to sleep, headaches and tension pains in the muscles.

These patients may receive complex hospital tests for physical disease without the real psychological nature of their problem being realized. Commonly they are investigated for hyperthyroidism or rare adrenal tumours. Sometimes they even undergo surgical operations (sympathectomy) to reduce their excessive perspiration.

The drug treatment described for phobias is also of value for the other types of anxiety state that we have mentioned. Diazepam 5 mg or chlordiazepoxide 10 mg three times daily relieves the average patient, both from the subjective feeling of apprehension and from the physical symptoms of anxiety. If it is the physical symptoms (such as palpitations) that are mainly troublesome then a drug may be used that blocks the activity of that part of the sympathetic nervous system (β-adrenergic blockade) such as propranolol.

Another method of treatment is **psychotherapy**. *Supportive* *psychotherapy* (see p. 164) is comforting and lowers the anxiety levels. This may give temporary relief to the patient, which in some cases is all that is necessary while waiting for the anxiety state to clear up with the passage of time (as most of them do). If the patient is subject to recurring attacks of anxiety then *insight-oriented* psychotherapy (see p. 168) should be considered. This is designed to get to the psychological roots of the problem. It has the drawbacks that it is a lengthy and expensive process, and that the insights that it produces may themselves temporarily **increase** the level of anxiety. Candidates for this type of treatment have to be carefully selected, therefore, and have to show a degree of strength of personality, perseverance and motivation, before being accepted for therapy.

Obsessional states

To understand obsessional states it is important to distinguish between a neurotic illness and a neurotic personality. An **illness** is diagnosed on the presence of symptoms: an abnormal personality is diagnosed on the basis of character traits. There are three main differences between character traits and symptoms.

Firstly not all of us have symptoms but we all have character traits. We are all, to different degrees, habitually conscientious, energetic, attention-seeking, tidy, talkative, or selfish. In describing an individual's personality we may say that he is conscientious, shy, and talkative. The conscientiousness, shyness and talkativeness are his **character traits**.

Secondly character traits alter little with the passage of time. Usually if we meet someone after many years he is still recognizably the same personality. Symptoms tend to be more transient.

Thirdly most people accept their own personalities. Symptoms, on the other hand, are usually distressing and unacceptable.

We can now distinguish between the obsessional personality and the obsessional illness. The **obsessional personality** shows the following character traits:

1   Orderliness. The person is typically punctual, clean, tidy, particular, fastidious and conscientious.

2   Obstinacy. For example he is stubborn and difficult to change in his views.

3 A tendency to hoard. He may be keen at collecting coins or stamps; or he may be mean and stingy – reluctant to part with money itself.

We can now consider the **obsessional state** – an illness that we can diagnose by its symptoms, which are as follows:

1 Rituals

The patient has to do things in a particular order, or a certain number of times. For example some individuals have to put their clothes on in the same order each day. Others have to wash their hands, say, three times every time they wash at all.

2 Doubts

Obsessional doubts make the patient wonder if something really happened – something that he was sure he saw or heard or felt. This may make him check excessively. Did he **really** lock the front door? He may have to go back many times to see that he really did. If he has this symptom together with a ritual he may take hours, for instance, to get dressed. If, towards the end of his dressing ritual, he thinks 'Did I really put my left sock on before the right sock' he may have to start all over again.

3 Ruminations

These are thoughts that go round and round in the patient's mind. Even if he finds them obscene, violent or distressing he is unable to keep them out of his mind.

4 Obsessional phobias

A mother may be afraid of knives, because she thinks she might kill her baby. This is slightly different from the phobic anxiety (in which there was merely a passive apprehension of experiencing something). In the obsessional phobia the patient usually has a fear that he will do something wrong against his better judgement. Obsessional symptoms may be seen as a way of repressing unacceptable thoughts or wishes, e.g. handwashing symbolizing the patient wishing to rid himself of unconscious guilt.

To diagnose a symptom as obsessional, the following three features should be present:

(a) The patient realizes that the feeling, thought or action is

irrational, with a subjective feeling of compulsion.
(b)   He has tried to resist it.
(c)   Resistance leads to an increase in tension or anxiety.

Minor degrees of obsessional symptoms are common and often require no treatment. In more severe degrees various treatments may be tried. Major tranquillizers (such as phenothiazines – see p. 140) may be helpful when given in large doses. Tricyclic antidepressants help some patients, and clomipramine is one used especially in obsessional states. There is often a mixture of depressive symptoms with the obsessional features, and ECT may relieve both in severe and incapacitating illness.

The usual forms of psychotherapy often fail, but **behaviour therapy** has been used with success in this situation. For those cases which are severe, distressing and long lasting, and which fail to respond to any other treatment, stereotactic brain surgery (p. 157) should be considered. Although it is rare for patients to need this, it can provide a relief, especially for those patients who are also continually tense and anxious.

HYSTERIA

The term hysteria is used in many different ways, which is confusing. To clarify this situation we shall start by separating the hysterical illness from the hysterical personality (on the same lines as we did for obsessional states).

The illness is diagnosed in the presence of **hysterical symptoms**:

(a)   Conversion symptoms. These mimic effects of physical illness, so that the patient might complain of paralysis, loss of the power of speech (aphonia), loss of sensation in the skin (anaesthesia), or difficulty with hearing or seeing (hysterical deafness or blindness).

(b)   Dissociation symptoms. Here the patient behaves as if the brain is not functioning properly, and complains of loss of memory, fits, faints or other disturbances of consciousness.

With both conversion and dissociation symptoms it is found that the patient, by developing the symptom, ends up by avoiding a situation of unbearable anxiety; this advantage granted by the symptom is called the **primary gain**. Sometimes the physician can tell from examining the patient that the symptoms and signs do not fit any common physical illness. This is a poor way of diagnosing hysteria, though, and it is better to base the diagnosis on a review of the patient's life situation that clearly shows up the primary gain or loss of anxiety accompanying the symptom.

For instance, a patient under persistent mental stress at his job may suddenly develop paralysed legs so that he can no longer get to work. The person who has experienced a calamitous disaster in his private life may wander off, lose his memory, and turn up in another town not knowing who he is.

The patient does not deliberately say to himself that he is going to lose his memory or stop moving his legs (consciously **pretending** to have an illness would be known as **malingering**). The patient with hysterical paraplegia, for instance, is not lying – he really cannot move his legs even though they are physically in full working order. Developing a hysterical symptom is a process that can happen to any normal person, under severe stress. Imagine a soldier in the front line, under constant fire, shooting his rifle in perpetual fear of losing his own life. If the tension becomes unbearable, he may suddenly find that his right arm is paralysed – maybe after a slight jolt. No matter how hard he **tries** to move the arm, he is unable to do so. It is as if something has snapped in his unconscious mind, and it is somehow better to have a paralysed arm than to stay there firing his rifle.

Hysterical personality

This is diagnosed from the presence of **hysterical personality traits.** The affected person may be attention-seeking, over-dramatic (histrionic), vain, talkative and egocentric. In his first approach to you he will possibly be excessively pleasant, charming and generally seductive. His behaviour is capable of sudden change, so that he becomes cold, indifferent or even hostile, indicating the initial superficiality of his warmth. Hysterical personalities often **manipulate** others: that is to say, they try to get their own way by devious means. They may use the charming approach just mentioned, or they may raise the anxieties of people in their environment by using veiled threats (e.g. of suicide). Although we used the pronoun 'he' just now, the hysterical personality is more often recognized among women than in men. This may be because in our society men are more directly aggressive, but a woman is expected to 'twist you round her little finger'. Of course, many of the character traits are acceptable in a child of four or five; the adult showing them is sometimes said to be fixated at this stage of development (the Oedipus complex – see p. 87). Defence mechanisms used by these persons include excessive repression and denial.

You will remember that in the hysterical illness the term **primary gain** was used to describe the loss of anxiety. Hysterical personalities often obtain a number of other advantages from their behaviour – these are known as **secondary gains**.

Treatment

The hysterical illness is a response to stress, and when the patient is removed from the anxiety provoking situation the symptoms often resolve within a few days. After that he can be given advice and help in dealing with his problems.

If the symptoms do not clear up of their own accord, it may be dangerous to make strenuous efforts to get rid of them. The story is told of a man who was admitted to hospital with paralysed legs, and who was given intensive hypnosis to get rid of his hysterical disability. He recovered, and then walked to the window and threw himself out. The point of this story is that a hysterical symptom may be merely a crude way of dealing with anxiety, but it may be the only way open to the patient. The anxiety may be overwhelming if he is suddenly required to come face to face with it.

What can be done is to allow the patient the opportunity to talk about himself. The conversation should be steered away from arguments about whether his paralysis is 'real', and on to his general life situation. Although at first he may deny that he has any serious problems, as his confidence grows he may be able gradually to call them to mind. Talking them over with the therapist often enables the patient to see them in a less nightmarish light, or to find some other way of coping with them less unrealistic than the hysterical symptom.

In other cases the patient is found to be suffering from a more serious mental illness. There the hysterical symptom is just the tip of the iceberg, and the underlying condition needs treatment or investigation.

Turning now to the hysterical personality, in most cases this is left untreated. Many such persons are able to use their character traits to financial or emotional advantage. A film starlet, for instance, may find that her natural ability to act and her ability to produce tears at the drop of a hat are great assets. Her vanity ensures that she makes herself look as attractive as possible. Her charm ensures she gets good parts. Her attention-seeking behaviour ensures publicity. Of course the defects of the hysterical personality may impair the quality of her private life.

The patient who strongly desires to have a radical change in his personality may be considered for psychoanalysis (see p. 168) but this method of treatment is expensive and time-consuming so that at present only a tiny minority of patients avail themselves of it.

An important problem occurs when a person with a hysterical personality develops a new physical illness. They are often wrongly diagnosed or they may antagonize the hospital staff. They are difficult to diagnose because they frequently exaggerate their symptoms, or behave in an over-dramatic (histrionic) way. These same traits, and their attention seeking behaviour, often produce a hostile reaction from the staff, who prefer a more brave 'stiff upper lip' approach. Their symptoms may be dismissed as just 'neurotic' or 'hysterical'.

Correct management can make a big difference to the outcome in this situation. If the garrulous patient is allowed to have his say, or if the patient screaming in 'intense agony' is told that the staff realize he is in great pain, then these sufferers do not need to go on proving their distress and they relax and are able to cooperate better. Of course, one can see that if the staff believe that the patient is being unnecessarily dramatic, then their cold response will only per-petuate the situation. Sensing the lack of sympathy, the patient will continue to talk at great length to make sure you understand his symptoms completely, or will continue to scream and roll about to make quite certain you take his pain seriously. By this stage the doctor or nurse is irritated and it is difficult for them to swallow their pride and do the only thing that will break through this vicious circle – to express serious concern to the patient about his predicament.

Hysteria is a common source of misdiagnosis. Hysterical illnesses may be falsely attributed to a patient with physical disease but few signs or misleading ones are present. Hysterical illness is often diagnosed when in fact physical illness is present (e.g. appendicitis) because of histrionic behaviour – screaming, shouting, demanding, exaggerating etc.; paralysis or loss of sensation (frequently diag-nosed as 'hysterical') may be part of a more serious mental illness (schizophrenia or organic brain disease).

In general, in order to avoid errors, hysterical symptoms should be carefully evaluated in terms of:

1 The form they take.
2 The setting in which they occur.
3 The gain to the patient.

Hysteria must be a positive diagnosis, not merely a diagnosis of exclusion.

DEPRESSIVE NEUROSIS

Depressive illness is one of the commonest conditions diagnosed by psychiatrists today. Some of these illnesses are of neurotic degree, and some psychotic. To describe a depression as a neurosis means:

1 It is more severe than a normal reaction to loss or dis-appointment.
2 It is not such a severe depression that one would call it a psychosis.

To satisfy the first rule we use the same criterion as we had for anxiety states – the depressive reaction is out of proportion to the cause, and is therefore **excessive in duration or degree**. We would call the illness a psychosis under the second rule if the patient suffered from delusions, hallucinations or gross abnormality of behaviour (e.g. sitting motionless for days or weeks).

There are two other terms that may need explanation – **endogenous** and **reactive**. A *reactive depression* is one which follows clearly upon a psychological stress (or series of stresses). An *endogenous depression* is one in which there is no obvious environmental cause (endogenous means 'arising from within'). Neurotic depressions tend to be reactive, whereas psychotic depressions are often endogenous, but there are many exceptions:

	Reactive	Endogenous
Neurotic	+ + + +	+ +
Psychotic	+ +	+ + + +

The events that trigger off a depressive illness are similar to those that might give rise to ordinary degrees of depression. They include bereavement (especially loss of spouse), the loss of other persons whether from death or from departure to a far off place, the loss of physical things that are loved (possessions), or the loss of more abstract things such as status and occupation. Loss of **role** can bring about depression. For instance, a woman married to a difficult and unpleasant husband, who obtained most of her satisfaction in life from bringing up and looking after her children, may become very depressed when her children are old enough to leave home, leaving her with just the husband to think about and cope with.

These are examples of depression arising from losses, separations or disappointments, but depression can also arise when aggression and hatred is bottled up and turned against oneself. To illustrate this let us examine the normal reaction to bereavement, which is one of grief. After a loved one dies, there often follows a period of numbness when the pain or grief is pushed to one side or forgotten. There is then intense sadness, accompanied by a preoccupation with thoughts about the dead person. A widow may even believe that she can see or hear her dead husband at times (this is one of the circumstances in which a hallucination does not indicate a psychosis – another instance occurs when someone is falling off to sleep and hears voices or sees visions). The widow goes through the process of mourning, thinking and grieving about times past. She usually expresses her grief emotionally by crying, sleeping poorly and eating without interest. Gradually this passes off and she recovers. This process proceeds naturally if the dead person was loved by the survivor. If there was no interest at all, then there will be little reaction. If relationships were completely hostile, the reaction may be one of relief or frank pleasure.

Let us take the case now where the relationship was **ambivalent**, that is to say that there was a fairly even mixture of love and hate. After the husband's death the numbness that the widow experiences continues for a long time. She finds it difficult to express grief. It is as if she cannot think about all the good things that happened without also thinking about all the bad things, which would be too painful to bear. So she does not go through the stage of mourning the loss, of feeling sad, of being preoccupied with the dead person. She rapidly resumes life in a way which, on the surface, seems much as before. Eventually, however, events catch up on her. After some months the hostile feelings start welling up inside her. This happened when her husband was alive, but then she was able to deal with them by thinking about his charm, his good looks or his occasional kindness. Now it is more difficult to deal with the hostility, and it tends to get turned inwards, so that she becomes guilty and self-critical and neglects herself.

Symptoms of depressive illness

There are certain central symptoms which are typical of depressive illness, whether it is neurotic or psychotic, reactive or endogenous (see also pp. 32–34).

Firstly the **mood** is depressed. The patient is sad, low in spirits or melancholy. It is sometimes the case that a patient will have all the other features of a depressive illness and not admit to *feeling* depressed, but this is not usual.

Secondly the **energy** and **behaviour** are affected. The patient feels weary, slowed up, and not inclined to do anything. In some cases this is obvious to the outside observer – the patient moves slowly, talks slowly, and there is a long gap before he answers a question. This slowing up is known as **retardation**. Even if it is not obvious to outsiders the patient is all too painfully aware of the feeling of being slowed up, of lacking energy or that everything is a great effort. The lack of energy affects mental function as well as physical effort, and depression brings about absentmindedness, difficulty with memory, and impaired concentration.

Thirdly there is a *loss of interest*. The patient is not interested in food, sex or making friends. He cannot be bothered doing anything or going anywhere. It seems as if the loss of interest is the factor that underlies the loss of energy – normally we have most energy for those things that are of greatest interest to us. If we have no interest at all, then where can we get the energy from?

Fourthly the thought processes are distorted. The patient looks on the black side of things. He is unduly pessimistic about the future, and even gives a gloomy account of his past. He tends to withdraw his interest from the world around him and have thoughts only about himself. Since they are gloomy thoughts they are likely to be about:

(a) The possibility that he may have diseases (hypochondriasis).
(b) Financial difficulties (often exaggerated).
(c) Guilt and self-criticism.
(d) Events that make him seem worthless or give him a low self-esteem.

Feeling that whatever they may do is likely to be wrong, such patients become indecisive, and complain of a loss of confidence.

Suicidal feelings may occur. Some patients will kill themselves before even seeking advice. However, even of those who commit suicide, the majority have tried to seek medical help, and presumably have felt disappointed or have been ignored. Others make a suicidal attempt (sometimes serious, sometimes trivial).

It seems reasonable to assume that patients like this have felt not only hopeless but also desperate. Some depressed patients make suicidal plans but do not carry them out. Others think of suicide, but only in vague terms. Some have strong moral or ethical reasons for not taking active steps to end their own lives, but would admit that they often go to bed feeling they wouldn't care if they didn't wake up.

Treatment

One can try to remove the cause of the depression, or one can try to help the patient to alter his attitude towards the cause.

Often the first of these remedies is not possible (e.g. with bereavement). Sometimes the patient can be helped to remedy the situation: for instance, if the patient is unhappily married, either a reconciliation or a trial separation may help. The therapist has to be very careful here: such suggestions may be a dangerous interference in a delicately balanced situation, and the patient may follow his advice with disastrous results. One should always beware of suggesting the **obvious solution**: if it is so obvious, why hasn't it been used before? Often it conflicts with important features of the patient's personality or value system, and he was right **not** to have taken that line. The patient who does not adopt the obvious solution because he is mentally handicapped or stupid enough not to be aware of it is a rarity.

On the other side of the coin, some patients can be assisted to take obvious steps to deal with their problems. They **see** the solution well enough, but the depression has so sapped their optimism, energy, enthusiasm and ability to cope that they do not have the confidence to **try** to do anything themselves. It is very worthwhile helping these patients to get out of this vicious circle of inability-to-deal-with-problems leading to depression, in turn leading to even greater inability-to-deal-with-problems.

How can we alter the attitudes of those whose problems are insuperable, or whose excessive depression is a result of irretrievable losses and disappointments? Often such patients are helped by talking about their situation. That is to say, the therapist listens to them; when they pause, he gets them to go on ('tell me some more about that') and occasionally shows them he has been listening ('that must have been a particularly bad time for you'). We do not understand completely why some patients get so much relief from 'getting it off their chest' or technically **ventilation** of their difficulties. It may be that actually putting them into words cuts down the distorted problems (that are such nightmarish giants in their imagination) into ordinary life size proportions.

Apart from these and other methods of supportive psychotherapy (see p. 164), **physical methods** of treatment may also be used. A general account of their action now follows but the details of their use will be found elsewhere (pp. 138–158).

Physical methods of treatment

In the past, stimulants (such as amphetamines) were used for treating depression. Although these made the patient feel more cheerful and active while he took them, as each dose wore off there was a nasty let-down. Some patients took more and more, and addiction became a problem.

With the coming of the **tricyclic antidepressants** the situation changed. These drugs are not pep pills – they have little or no effect on patients that are not depressed to start with. They are remarkably free from addictive action. The term 'tricyclic' derives from the basic chemical formulae (see below), which are similar to that of the phenothiazines (see p. 140).

Imipramine group	Amitriptyline group	Phenothiazines
R	R	N R

These drugs are used in both neurotic and psychotic types of depression. They tend to be more effective in endogenous than in reactive depression – clearly if the patient lives in a permanently depressive environment then not too much can be expected of pills. Moreover, it is found that the most rapid results are obtained with those cases in which symptoms such as **loss of weight** and **early morning waking** are prominent – features that are found more often with the endogenous type of depression. Nevertheless, even when these 'endogenous' features are absent, and obvious objective stresses are conspicuous, there may still be an even chance of success with these drugs. For instance, some patients with inoperable cancer will feel much better on them.

If they do prove successful, it is worth taking them for some months. The benefit usually becomes obvious within about ten days of the start of a regular course, and further improvement occurs for a month or more. In these cases it has been shown that patients who at this stage continue to take the active medication relapse far less frequently than patients who are switched to identical looking placebo tablets.

Most of these drugs (e.g. imipramine, amitriptyline, nortriptyline, protriptyline, dothiepin) have a tendency to block the action of the parasympathetic nervous system. The atropine-like side effects that result are dry mouth, blurred vision and constipation. They should be used cautiously, if at all, for patients with closed angle glaucoma or prostatic hypertrophy.

If any of these side effects prove troublesome the dose of the drug should be reduced – there is a very wide variation in the amount that patients require.

Disorders of cardiac conduction or rhythm are a hazard in acute overdosage, or in those on long term therapy who suffer some trauma to the heart muscle (e.g. from myocardial infarction). Tricyclics impair the action of peripherally acting hypotensive. drugs (probably through inhibition of uptake of the hypotensive drug into its site action in the sympathetic nerve ending), so that the treatment of combined hypertension and depressive illness requires special care. On the whole these drugs have otherwise proved to be relatively safe. Further aspects of their use are considered in the chapter on treatment (Chapter 17).

The monoamine oxidase inhibitors (MAOIs) form a quite different group of antidepressant drugs. In the central nervous system impulses are conveyed from one neurone to the next by means of chemical transmitters (amines), which include noradrenaline and 5-hydroxytryptamine (5HT, serotonin). The nerve impulses are more frequent if the amount of amine present is increased, thus increasing the activity of that part of the nervous system. Normally the amines disappear from the nerve junction:

(a)   Through re-uptake back into the nerve cells from which they were released.

(b)   Through destruction by the enzyme monoamine oxidase.

The tricyclic antidepressants block method (a), and the MAOIs block method (b). There have been some hazards in the clinical use of MAOIs. They block the destruction that normally takes place of some drugs, and of some naturally occurring amines in foodstuffs. Tyramine, present in cheese, accumulates and causes a dangerous rise of blood pressure under these circumstances, and the patient may die from cerebral haemorrhage (e.g. from an unsuspected arterial aneurysm).

Other methods of physical treatment include electroconvulsive therapy (ECT) and brain surgery. ECT is used in serious cases of depression, for instance when the patient is actively suicidal. It acts more quickly than drugs. Its use is considered more fully elsewhere (p. 151). Brain surgery (leucotomy, stereotactic surgery) is rarely used for uncomplicated depressive illness, but may be considered in those unfortunate cases that fail to improve with ordinary methods of management, and which give rise to severe long-standing tension and distress (p. 156)

The suicidal patient

Suicide (the completed act) is distinguished from attempted suicide. In England the suicide rate is slowly falling, but hospital admissions from drug overdoses have risen to alarming proportions.

Taking first, then, those persons that actually kill themselves, who are they likely to be? Typically they are men more often than women, old rather than young, and of high social class (often with recent loss of money, status or role). They tend to be living alone (not currently married) in the centre of a city, and they often have a history of conflict with the law, alcoholism or drug dependence, or a psychiatric history of depression or schizophrenia.

This is just a picture built up from the known statistics, but there are people who kill themselves who show none of these characteristics. Are there better ways of judging who is at risk? There are two indicators that are much more important than any of these factors.

The first is the subject's own statement. If he says that he feels like killing himself, this should be taken seriously. There used to be a myth that those people that spoke of it never did it. This idea is quite wrong. In fact a person who admits to serious thoughts about suicide may be ten, twenty or even a hundred times as likely to kill himself as the next man.

The second pointer is a recent episode of attempted suicide. The suicide rate in the year following an attempt may be a hundred or even two hundred times as great as in the average population.

When a patient takes an overdose of drugs, this is sometimes dismissed as a mere 'gesture'. There is, no doubt, often a desire on the part of the patient to seek attention or to manipulate the feelings and actions of other people. Such patients do not seem to be in the suicidal category at first sight. They are often young, female and from the lower social classes (in contrast to the classical picture presented above). However, the reader will now appreciate that any patient that attempts suicide should not be dismissed too lightly. On the contrary, if one wishes to cut down the number of deaths from suicide, this is one population on which it would be worth concentrating.

Management of the suicidal patient

In the past doctors were afraid to ask patients openly if they were suicidal, for fear of putting the idea into their heads. It is now realized that it is far more dangerous not to give the patient a chance to express his feelings.

Patients kill themselves when they feel:

(a) Hopeless.
(b) Desperate.

It is when these feelings are present **together** that the danger exists. It is therefore reasonable always to ask the patient 'Do you ever feel that there is no hope?' and later in the interview 'Do you ever feel like doing something desperate?' If you feel able to do so without embarrassment you may ask the patient 'Do you ever seriously feel like killing yourself?' Some patients with strong moral or religious beliefs about the **wickedness** of the act of suicide will deny being aware of such feelings until it is too late. For them an easier question is 'Do you go to sleep not caring whether you will wake up?'.

If the patient has suicidal thoughts he should be encouraged to talk about his feelings. Allow him to express how hopeless he sees the outlook to be, and how he despairs at times. Overdoses are ways of **acting out** problems: one of the principles of psychotherapy is that patients who can **talk out** their problems no longer need to act them out.

If a patient thinks that no-one believes him, and that no-one understands how low he feels, he may be tempted in his despair to **show** them. If he can communicate in words the depth of his agony, he does not feel the need to convince you in other ways. Moreover, he may even feel that you care.

The danger in asking someone about his suicidal feelings is in briefly exposing their presence and then proceeding to talk about something else as if you hadn't heard or were not bothered about the way he felt. If you treat his feelings with respect and concern he is unlikely to resent you asking, and may even be grateful. Many inexperienced therapists are worried about encouraging patients to talk about their suicidal feelings. Partly they shrink away from coming face to face with someone else's stark misery, but they are also in difficulties because they do not know how to end their interview after the patient has finished expressing his pessimistic views. Similar difficulties are met with in talking to patients after they have taken an overdose.

In fact there is usually no need to end the interview by giving the patient profound insights into his problems, nor even by wholesale reassurance. **It is often enough just to say that you will see him again soon and talk about it some more**. This leaves the prospect of hope still alive, and allows him to believe that someone cares. The majority of patients will feel quite differently about life within a few weeks.

It is current hospital policy that all patients who have been admitted for attempted suicide should be seen by a psychiatrist. Feelings of hopelessness expressed by the patient are frequently the reason for a general practitioner referring that patient to a psychiatric clinic.

To summarize, the patient should be encouraged to reveal his suicidal thoughts, and allowed to talk about his hopelessness and despair. He should be supported by repeated interviews and prompt psychiatric referral in most cases.

The majority of depressed patients can be helped over the more despairing phase of their condition with these simple measures. When, at a particular time, a patient is expressing serious suicidal intent, admission as an inpatient to a psychiatric unit as a matter of emergency, even compulsorily (p. 121), will have to be considered.

For most patients an overdose is an isolated event. For a minority it is repeated again and again, with several admissions to hospital over a few years or even months. This repeated suicidal behaviour is less likely to be associated with a severe depressive illness but more likely to be a sign of personality disorder (see p. 3). Such patients, although typically young, will often give a history of antisocial acts or other evidence of difficulties in interpersonal relationships. They are certainly at risk, and may end up killing themselves, but they are very difficult to help.

4 Affective Disorders

The **affective (or emotional) disorders** are a group of illnesses which fit into a continuum between sadness and excessive cheerfulness, and in which the mood state or affect is the fundamental disturbance leading to the development of many other symptoms. They comprise:

1   The anxiety states (see Chapter 3). They have a controversial place in this group of disorders. They are regarded by many authorities as being separate illnesses, and not part of the affective disorders, despite their close relationship to mood changes.

2   Depressive neurosis (see Chapter 3).

3   Manic depressive psychosis. An illness in which discrete episodes of depression and mania or hypomania are found, or alternating episodes of these two extremes of mood.

4   Involutional melancholia.

The classification of depression

Depression as an affect may be defined as the subjective feeling of sadness, unhappiness, despondency, gloom or misery.

In Chapter 3, it has been pointed out that depression, for example following bereavement and loss of recognition of self-esteem (failing an examination, losing a job or a disappointment in love), occurs as:

1   The normal reaction to a common stress

In this instance, it is not usually severe, is short lived, self-limiting, and recovery is followed by a return to normal life. This type of reaction occurs commonly in most people at some period in their lives. It is often difficult to locate the precise point in time when this type of depression becomes pathological.

Grief reactions are an important and common 'normal' reaction to loss. The loss may be real, e.g. the loss of a loved one. Quite frequently it is the response to an imagined or even a symbolic event.

In other situations, the grief may be delayed for weeks or months because of attempts at supporting the morale of others or a desire to avoid the spectacle of mourning.

The typical features of grief reactions are intense feelings of anguish and sorrow and an obsessional preoccupation with the deceased.

Feelings of guilt concerning the relationship develop and there is frequently hostility towards friends and relatives. Apathy and 'exhaustion' then develop.

If this sequence of events is prolonged for more than several months, it is regarded as being pathological.

Insidiously, the depression may deepen and develop psychotic features. Suicidal thoughts or attempts frequently complicate the illness at this point.

2 Depressive neurosis (reactive or neurotic depression) (see Chapter 3).

As has been discussed, this is more severe, prolonged in time, dominating the individual's life and thoughts, is often progressive in severity and is usually **related to precipitating stress**. Personality traits of vulnerability, hypersensitivity, and neurotic conflicts with a low tolerance for stress are often present.

3 The depressive phase of the manic depressive psychosis

This is usually referred to as **endogenous depression** and implies that there are no obvious environmental precipitating causes.

In fact, clinically, this is rarely the case: precipitating causes are often present, and there may be a significant overlay of neurotic symptoms, rendering it difficult to distinguish from a depressive neurosis, especially if the latter is severe.

In general, the patient's personality cannot be separated from his depressive illness and the two are intimately bound together.

Leonhard in 1959 described:

(a) Unipolar depression – in which mania or hypomania never occurs. This group included involutional melancholias in older patients.

(b)   Bipolar depression – which he regarded as the true manic depressive illness, in which both phases, depression and mania, ultimately occurred. Only 20% – 25% of cases of endogenous depression fit into this group.

4   Involutional melancholia

Is regarded by some authorities as a discrete illness and by others as endogenous (in particular agitated) depression occurring in the involutional period.

Another view is that **all depressions fit on a continuum from mild to severe**. This has practical significance in that severe depressive neurosis as well as 'endogenous' depression may be responsive to ECT (electroconvulsive therapy). Also, it is frequently very difficult to distinguish between a mild endogenous depression, in which perhaps personality factors and environmental stress are involved, and a reactive type depression.

The natural history of depression and mania is shown in Fig. 1. With both depression and mania, there may be long periods of remission in between attacks.

It should be noted too, that an individual may develop a depressive neurosis at one point in time, and at another an endogenous type depression.

The symptoms of depression have been discussed in Chapter 3. The series of symptoms that are characteristic of the endogenous depressive syndrome are as follows:

1(a)   Mental and physical 'slowing up' of thought and movement which may progress to the point of **psychomotor retardation**. In more severe cases, a **depressive stupor** with total loss of interest in the environment and **mutism** develops.

1(b)   Other cases present with varying degrees of **agitation, restlessness** and **anxiety**.

2   Self-reproach, brooding about the past, indecisiveness and feelings of a loss of self-esteem and self-confidence.

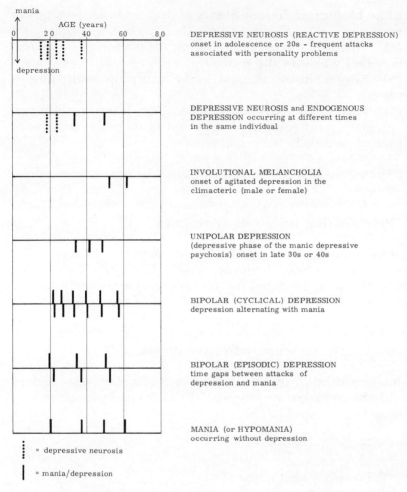

Fig. 1 The natural history of depression and the manic depressive psychosis

3 Depressive ideas verging on the delusional, or frankly delusional, may be present. Most frequently they are **delusions of sin, disease, unworthiness, hypochondriasis and poverty**. They indicate that the depression has reached **psychotic proportions**.

4 Paranoid ideas may develop.

5 Suicidal thoughts are very common and must be taken seriously.

6   The biological concomitants of depression are present, for example:

(a)   There is a **diurnal mood swing** and patients complain that they **feel worse in the morning**.

(b)   **Severe insomnia** and **early morning wakening** is present.

(c)   There is a **loss of libido**, constipation, **loss of weight and appetite**, and frequently a reduction in the pulse rate, blood pressure and body temperature.

7   There is frequently a previous or family history of depression or hypomania.

8   Precipitating stress may be absent.

9   Obsessional and **hysterical** symptoms or character traits sometimes complicate depressive illness. The depression acts as a catalyst allowing the dormant personality characteristics to become exposed so that they form an integral part of the clinical picture.

10   A mixture of schizophrenic type symptoms with depression or elation is termed a **schizo–affective illness**.

It is important to appreciate that depression may be **secondary to other psychiatric or physical illness**. It may be the presenting symptom of:

(a)   Organic disease, e.g.:
        A brain tumour
        Following a viral illness
        Endocrine illness
        Addisons disease
        Myasthenia gravis
        Cerebral syphilis
(b)   Other psychiatric illness, e.g.:
        Schizophrenia
        It may also complicate personality disorder or subnormality.

The symptoms of mania and hypomania

Hypomania is the term used to describe the milder forms of mania.

They represent the elated phase of the manic depressive psychosis.

The illness has a wide range of severity varying from mild hypomania to severe manic excitement.

Both mania and hypomania are far less frequently diagnosed than depression, and the bipolar variation is uncommon (see Fig. 2).

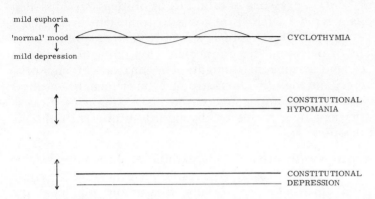

Fig. 2 Constitutional mood tendencies which may lead to manic depressive psychosis

Predisposed individuals (for depression and mania) often describe life-long mild mood swings from mild depression to mild euphoria. This is the **cyclothymic personality.** Other patients are persistently mildly depressed (constitutional depressives) and others mildly euphoric, filled with energy and excessively driving in their activities (constitutionally hypomanic).

The **onset of symptoms** may be sudden or develop over a period of days or weeks (depression as well as mania).

The clinical picture comprises 4 groups of symptoms:

1   A mood change varying from mild euphoria and expansive cheerfulness to excitement and unrestrained elation.

Lability of mood is frequently present, and the excited euphoric patient inexplicably lapses into tearful sadness.

The keynote of the mood change is the **infectious optimism** which is so readily communicated to observers, and the unrealistic grandiosity of the patient's plans that accompany it.

2   Motor activity is increased, the patient becoming restless, overactive and agitated, eventually to the point of exhaustion. Behaviour, as a whole, is exaggerated and the individual is importunate, demanding and interfering, talking loudly or shouting frequently.

3   Thought processes are increased. Thinking becomes more rapid and there is a **pressure of talk**. **Flight of ideas** develops: that is, there is a rapid switch from topic to topic which is often a response to a verbal or perceptual cue – noises and the presence and movement of objects in the immediate environment serving to initiate a rapid change in thought. The mixture of euphoria, distractability and flight of ideas introduces an element of wittiness and the use of puns into conversation. When flight of ideas is extreme it may be difficult to distinguish from schizophrenic thought disorder.

4   Psychotic symptoms include grandiose and paranoid delusions (in 40% – 50% of cases). As a result, the patient may become involved in financially or socially disasterous schemes, the implausability of which only become obvious when it is too late. Other patients have the conviction that they are God or Jesus. Secondary paranoid delusions may occur (see Chapter 6).

Auditory hallucinations develop in about 10% of cases and are also grandiose in nature, for example, hearing the voice of God.

Patients may become paranoid, interfering, dogmatic, hyperactive and excitable **without** developing frank psychotic symptoms.In others, sexual and moral disinhibition predominate.

In keeping with the severity of the illness, a degree of **insight and judgement is always lost.**

Acute mania has to be differentiated from catatonic (schizophrenic) excitement. In the former, hallucinations are rare, good rapport may be established, and the patient's mood is not flat, incongruous or remote. Negativism is rarely present and the behaviour, as a whole, is more organized and purposive. Typical schizophrenic thought disorder is absent (see Chapter 5).

Mania may also be simulated by the excitement of **amphetamine intoxication**. The presence of predominantly paranoid delusions, visual as well as auditory hallucinations and some clouding of consciousness in amphetamine intoxication, together with their presence in the blood and urine, establish the diagnosis.

Treatment

1 Depression

Most patients are treatable on an outpatient or day hospital basis. Hospitalization may be required if suicidal thoughts are present, or if the patient is retarded, severely agitated or self-neglectful.

Tricyclic antidepressants (imipramine and amitryptiline series) are the drugs of choice in 'endogenous type' depression. The dosage ranges up to 200–300 mg daily. They are effective in 60%–70% of cases within 4–8 weeks.

Administration of tricyclic antidepressants

The tricyclic antidepressants are extremely safe in the customary dosage but precautions can be taken against the more serious potential ill-effects. Suicidal talk or behaviour, or even small overdoses, should be taken seriously (see p. 26) since these drugs can be lethal in large quantities, e.g. by inducing cardiac arrhythmias. The last feature also contraindicates their use in recent myocardial infarction. A previous history (or family history) of epileptic seizures warns of the possibility of convulsions, the tendency to which these compounds increase. The patient should not drive or work with dangerous machinery until he has had a chance to assess how **drowsy** the tablets make him. This applies to all psychotropic drugs.

The tricyclic antidepressants may produce a variety of **minor side effects.** It is often difficult to separate the effects of the drug from the symptoms of the depression itself (e.g. tiredness, difficulty in concentration) or from the associated anxiety (tremor, sweating, palpitations, dizziness). The anxiety features may even worsen temporarily during the first few weeks of treatment as the patient is forced out of a position of resigned helplessness into active contact with reality.

One group of side effects that is characteristic of the tricyclics is the syndrome of **cholinergic blockade.** The action of the parasympathetic nervous system is inhibited, producing dry mouth, blurred vision and constipation or difficulty with micturition. These effects, though usually not serious, may be troublesome to the patient. In general they suggest that the dose may be reduced, or if this is not possible then symptomatic treatment (high fibre diet for constipation, frequent drinks for dry mouth) may be sufficient.

These tendencies do contraindicate the use of these compounds when the patient is known to suffer from glaucoma or prostatic hypertrophy. The action of tricyclic drugs tends to be antagonistic to that of antihypertensive drugs, so special care is needed in the patient who requires treatment for both depression and hypertension, and each patient must be considered individually.

Duration of treatment

If the patient responds well to the drug, and is not significantly bothered by side effects, how long should he continue to take it? In general one wishes to prescribe drugs for as short a time as possible, but there are drawbacks to immediate cessation of treatment as soon as the patient feels back to his old self. Relapse at this stage may not respond as well as the initial episode. Furthermore patients will tend to stop taking the tablets unless they are convinced of their value. If, back in depressive low spirits, he finds it difficult to recall that he ever **was** improved, he will not be very keen to go back on what he regards as useless medication.

It is therefore advisable to encourage the patient to continue taking the drug for weeks or months after recovery has taken place. He can be assured that he will not become 'addicted' to his tablets, since physical dependence is not a problem with this class of compound. It has been shown that the relapse rate is conspicuously increased in those who stop their tricyclic prematurely. After a month or two of normality, the patient himself will recognize the significance of any depressive symptoms that recur when the dose is eventually reduced, and will be motivated to return to the normal dosage until the time is ripe for a gradual but complete withdrawal. Unfortunately in the present state of knowledge choosing the right moment for this remains a matter of trial and error.

MAOIs (monoamine oxidase inhibitors) are effective in depressive neurosis, especially cases where phobic anxiety and hysterical features are present.

Combinations of the two groups of drugs are sometimes used in resistant depression, but this is thought by many psychiatrists to be dangerous.

Failure to respond to drug therapy indicates that **ECT** may be required. With ECT 8 or 10 treatments is the average course. The relapse rate is lower and the number required less when ECT is combined with tricyclics. Grossly retarded patients respond best to ECT. The presence of firm suicidal thoughts is a strong indication.

After recovery, antidepressant medication with tricyclics is continued for a minimum of 2–3 months to prevent relapses.

General nursing care, sympathetic supportive handling and listening to the patient are important adjuncts to the management of all patients who, if in hospital, will spend most of their time being cared for by the nursing staff.

Minor tranquillizers (diazepam or chlordiazepoxide) are given to relieve agitation and anxiety.

Major tranquillizers (phenothiazines such as chlorpromazine) are given if severe agitation and psychotic ideas are present.

Hypnotics may be necessary for persistent insomnia, e.g. chloral hydrate or nitrazepam (see p. 144).

Small doses of insulin by injection are occasionally given over a period of 2 weeks to stimulate the appetite of withdrawn, anorexic, apathetic patients who have lost a lot of weight.

Resistant cases of depression sometimes respond to a combination of L-tryptophan (from which the body manufactures serotonin) 2–4 g daily, with a MAOI drug such as Marplan or Nardil. This combination is more effective in depression which has basically neurotic or reactive elements. A small minority of cases unresponsive to drugs or ECT are submittable to **stereotactic surgery** (see Chapter 17).

Patients in hospital are encouraged to take part in occupational therapy (see p. 183).

2 Mania and hypomania

Most patients with hypomania need to be treated in a hospital setting because of their unpredictability, uncooperativeness and uninhibited sexual or spendthrift behaviour. They require rapid control with:

(a) Major tranquillizers, such as chlorpromazine orally or i.m. or thioridazine orally. In exceptionally severe excitement i.v. dosage is given. Oral doses vary from 300–1500 mg daily.

(b) Butyrophenones (e.g. haloperidol) may be given as an alternative, orally 8–80 mg daily, or 10–20 mg at a time i.m. or i.v. They are often combined with a phenothiazine. An antidote to their potential extrapyramidal side effects must always be at hand (i.m. or i.v. procyclidine hydrochloride).

(c) ECT may need to be given if the patient cannot be rapidly controlled with tranquillizers; 3 or 4 ECT on alternate days is an average requirement. Improvement after ECT is usually dramatic.

(d) Lithium preparations (0.25 g three times a day) are used in the acute state and then indefinitely in order to prevent relapses. A blood level of 0.5–1.5 mmol/l is maintained. There are many side effects and treatment must be under medical supervision (see p. 149).

(e) Night sedation is usually necessary.

Insight orientated **psychotherapy** is of little value in the acute phase of both depression and hypomania, but their treatment can be aided considerably by skilled management and support.

With recovery, personality problems and environmental stresses are explored and discussed.

Further details of drug treatment are considered in Chapter 17.

Aetiology of the manic depressive psychosis

The illness occurs at some time in the life of 10% or so of most populations with a prevalence of 3–4 per 1000 at any one time.

(a) It is more common in Jews and Mediterranean peoples.
(b) The sex ratio is 3:2 in favour of women.
(c) The premorbid personality is frequently cyclothymic (see Fig. 1).
(d) Many patients are **pyknic** (stocky, short limbed, stout, with large visceral cavities).

A hereditary factor is likely because of the frequent presence of a family history of affective disorder. In 10% of cases, one or other parent has had the illness. From 12.5 to 25% of the children of an affected parent and 20% of the siblings of an affected patient develop the illness. The incidence in identical twins (concordance rate) as opposed to non-identical twins, is extremely high (68% or more). There is no firm evidence that the illness is transmitted by a simple dominant or recessive gene. Multifactorial genetic inheritance is much more likely.

A physiological factor is probably involved. Supporting evidence for this is as follows:

(a) Mood changes are very commonly found in endocrine illness such as Cushing's syndrome, Addison's disease, myxoedema and thyrotoxicosis; also premenstrually, post-partum and in menopausal women.

(b) Many patients respond rapidly to ECT and antidepressant drugs.

(c) The illness is frequently precipitated by physical disease, especially viral, and drugs such as reserpine, sulphonamides and benzhexol.

(d) The periodicity of the illness suggests a biochemical basis.

(e) Electrolyte abnormalities have been demonstrated – specifically an abnormal movement of sodium chloride and potassium in and out of tissue and brain cells with sodium chloride retention. Treatment with lithium is thought to replace the sodium in the cells.

(f) Another theory is that the illness is due to reduction in available catecholamines at synapses in the CNS (central nervous system; see p. 148, e.g. reserpine lowers the catecholamine level (noradrenaline and serotonin) producing depression. MAOIs raise the catecholamine level curing depression by preventing the breakdown of catecholamines by MAO (monoamine oxidase).

(g) Pollitt has attributed the somatic changes of depression to a hypothalamic inbalance which he calls 'the functional depressive shift'.

Psychological factors. No single factor has been incriminated. Personality disorder, vulnerability and their relationship to environmental stress are important precipitating factors. Unresolved childhood conflicts, separation anxiety, delayed emotional development and life in a disorganized community, with lack of integration in a specific social group are other factors frequently quoted. The illness seems more common in urban as opposed to rural life where pressures are less evident.

Psychoanalytically, depression is regarded as the internalization of aggression, i.e. repression of a socially unacceptable wish producing exaggerated guilt feelings. Regression to an oral phase of psychosexual development occurs ('stage of dependency' – see p. 86).

Mania is seen as a 'defence' mechanism preventing the

production of depression, like 'whistling to keep one's spirits up'.

In primitive societies, the standard clinical picture of depression is uncommon. Hysterical, paranoid and hypochondriacal symptoms are more frequent and are probably depressive equivalents.

Involutional melancholia

This affective psychosis develops in the involutional period of life, between the ages of 45 and 65.

(a) It is more common in women in the ratio 3:1.
(b) There is a significant absence of previous affective or psychoneurotic illness.
(c) A premorbid personality with obsessional characteristics is often shown.

The typical features of psychotic depression, as described, develop with an accent on the following features:

1 Agitation, restlessness and anxiety frequently dominate the clinical picture.
2 Delusional ideas of guilt, worthlessness, nihilism, sin, disease and poverty occur.
3 Hypochondriacal ideas may antedate other symptoms and reach delusional intensity. Concern that the bowels are 'blocked' is very common.
4 Suicidal thoughts and self-reproach frequently occur. All melancholics must be regarded as potential suicidal risks.
5 Paranoid ideas, depersonalization and derealization are often associated.
6 The onset of the illness is usually gradual.

The response to treatment with ECT is so dramatic as to be diagnostic. Tricyclic antidepressants are very effective in less severe cases. The concept of involutional melancholia as a separate affective illness is questionable since any of the above features may occur in other depressive states.

Hypochondriasis

This is so frequently associated with affective disorders that it requires further discussion.

It is defined as 'the constant preoccupation with health together with an exaggerated concern with the real or imagined signs and symptoms of illness'.

Patients are difficult to reassure, either in respect of their claimed symptoms or their conviction that they are ill.

In the majority of cases in general practice (about 85%) hypochondriasis may be regarded as the somatic equivalent of depression or anxiety. It is, therefore, commonly associated with psychoneurotic disorders (especially depressive neurosis), psychotic depression, involutional melancholia and schizophrenia.

In about 15% cases there is an absence of emotional or other illness. The term **primary hypochondriasis** is reserved for this group.

Younger patients frequently present with single bizarre hypochondriacal complaints, for example the conviction that the face or nose is distorted in some way. A percentage of these cases are eventually diagnosed as schizophrenia or obsessional illness.

In the older individual, single or multiple specific or vague hypochondriacal complaints may continue for many years.

Conventional psychotherapy and drug treatment are of little avail and the patient becomes a familiar and importunate presence in medical, surgical and psychiatric clinics.

Recently it has been claimed that the neuroleptic drug pimozide may be successful when other neuroleptic drugs have failed.

5 Schizophrenia

That there is no ideal system of classification in psychiatry is well illustrated by the differing views concerning the concept of schizophrenia.

Schizophrenia is regarded as one of the **functional psychoses**, which implies a disorder with no demonstrable organic basis, at least in our present state of knowledge. Other examples of functional psychoses are the affective psychoses (manic depressive illness) and paranoid psychoses.

Schizophrenia is probably a **group of different syndromes** (that is, a collection of signs and symptoms, each with differing but overlapping features, a different prognosis and perhaps different causation) rather than a single discrete illness. Nevertheless, a general preliminary definition will be given.

Definition

Schizophrenia is a functional psychosis in which the symptoms are not understandable as an affective response. It is a syndrome in which specific psychological symptoms lead, in most cases, to disintegration and disorganization of the individual's personality. The symptoms interfere with thinking, emotion, motor behaviour and volition (will power), each in a characteristic way.

The abnormal thinking leads to misinterpretations of reality with the development of fantasy thinking, delusions and hallucinations. Insight is always lost to a variable degree.

Kraepelin, in 1896, differentiated it from the manic depressive psychosis, and described 3 basic types (paranoid, hebephrenic, catatonic). He coined the term 'dementia praecox' to describe the progression of the illness from its onset in adolescence to a dementing-like state in middle age. In 1861, **E. Bleuler** first used the term 'schizophrenia' and added a fourth type (simple schizophrenia) to Kraepelin's three basic types.

44

Langfeldt in 1911 introduced a new descriptive typology which is still widely used. He described:

1 Process schizophrenia, in which a relentless and progressive disintegration and deterioration of the personality occurs.

2 Reactive (schizophreniform) psychoses, where the onset of the illness seemed to be precipitated by environmental or emotional pressures, and in which the long term prognosis was relatively good.

Further reference to classification will be made after discussion of the signs and symptoms of the illness.

Incidence

The expectancy of an individual developing schizophrenia varies in different countries from 0.3 to 1.0%, probably due to diagnostic differences, or more rarely, inbreeding in isolated communities.

In most western European countries and the USA, the expectancy is about 0.85% and about 40% of chronic patients in mental hospitals are schizophrenic.

It is important to appreciate the point made originally by Bleuler that there are **latent** as well as **overt** schizophrenics. The former term is used to describe the large numbers of individuals who function indefinitely in the community with symptoms without ever being hospitalized, or indeed receiving psychiatric treatment of any kind.

Aetiology

How or why schizophrenia develops remains an enigma, despite extensive research. Current views indicate that it is most likely to be a breakdown in the balance between three interreacting sets of factors – **heredity, environmental and psychological stress**, and **physiological change**, possibly related to an inbalance of an enzyme or chemical factor in the brain. Some of these possibilities need to be examined in more detail:

Heredity

Twin studies seem to indicate that a genetic factor is certainly involved. The chance of an identical twin developing schizophrenia if his twin has it is 60% or more, whereas if the twins are non identical, the chances are no higher than for the rate between siblings (5–15%). These figures seem to hold true even in cases where the twins are separated at birth, therefore discounting the effect of the environment. The rate for schizophrenia in one or other of the parents of a schizophrenic child is 5–10%.

The mode of inheritance is probably through what is called **genetic heterogeneity**. That is, there are probably many genes involved, each exerting a small effect in different ways. This helps explain why schizophrenia occurs in childhood, adolescence and old age, and also the variations in its clinical forms.

In schizophrenia the percentage of children affected when one parent has the illness varies from 10 to 20%.

Environment

Attempts at relating schizophrenia to a wide variety of factors (e.g. age, sex, marital status, social class, location in town or country, degree of geographical mobility, native or foreign birth, religion, nationality and ethnic group) have been unconvincing.

Some studies have shown that it is more prevalent in areas of high social mobility and disorganization, especially in members of social class 5. These findings may be the result not the cause of schizophrenia, in that the personality changes produced by the illness render individuals more incompetent socially (see p. 136). Also, less deprived families tend to provide better care for their ill.

Psychological

Psychological factors, possibly acting on a genetic basis, have also been extensively studied.

Lidz has described situations in which a child withdraws from reality in order to defend itself from unresolved anxiety. This conflict may arise because of an inability in using one parent as a model to identify with, or as a love object, without antagonizing the other parent.

Bateson described similar conflicts in children exposed to a

double bind situation – where parents repeatedly say one thing and mean another.

The emotional deprivation resulting from the breakdown of the mother/child relationship where the mother is **'schizophrenogenic'** (cold, rejecting, obsessively anxious) has also been put forward as a possible important factor.

Children in the situation described find it difficult to relate to people, show little emotion at all, or an inappropriate one in a given situation, in an attempt at defending themselves from emotional stress. They find it difficult to make decisions or respond to the demands of others and avoid commitment in speech and tend to be evasive.

It is of interest that all these features fit into the pattern of the fundamental symptoms of schizophrenia (described later).

R. D. Laing attempts to explain schizophrenia as a situation in which families force a member into a position where he develops psychotic type behaviour as the only means of adapting to or coping with the abnormal family. In this sense, he does not regard the behaviour as a 'medical illness'.

Psychoanalysts see schizophrenia as a regression to an infantile 'auto-erotic' (narcisisstic self-preoccupation) level of thinking and behaviour due to the breakdown of their 'defence' mechanisms, in situations that have provoked severe emotional stress.

Prepsychotic personality

Many schizophrenics have traits (coldness, aloofness, slight emotional detachment and withdrawal from their environment) indicating that they had been **schizoid** personalities for many years before the development of formal symptoms. Others with these traits never develop schizophrenia.

The presence, in the same family, of normal children, a schizoid personality, a possible schizoid psychopathic personality and a frank schizophrenic, is further evidence of a multiple (polygenic) gene basis as a substrate for the illness, possibly interacting with environmental and psychological factors. For example, in a family with six children the following might be found:

1	2	3	4	5	6
normal	normal	normal	schizoid	schizoid psychopath	schizo-phrenic

Physical and biochemical factors

1 Kretschmer has shown that many schizophrenics are asthenic or 'ectomorphic', that is tall, lean, narrow chested.

2 Brain histology is normal.

3 There is no positive relationship to endocrine disorder with one exception – a syndrome **(Gjessing's)** wherein catatonic symptoms develop in association with nitrogen retention, thought to be due to abnormal thyroid metabolism. Improvement is said to occur rapidly after treatment with thyroxin and a low protein diet.

4 An aromatic fatty acid derivative, hexenoic acid, has been isolated in the sweat of chronic schizophrenics. It is related to the hormone in bees used to regulate ovarian growth in bee larvae. Its significance in man is not known.

5 There are non-specific 'epileptic-like' or slow waves in the electroencephalograph in 25% of patients. **Slater** has described a variety of schizophrenia developing 10–14 years after the onset of epilepsy in some patients.

6 Although biochemical investigations have been disappointing **a biochemical basis is nevertheless likely** because:

(a)   There is almost certainly a genetic factor involved.

(b)   No convincing psychological cause has yet been demonstrated, although this does not preclude the role of psychological factors in the precipitation of the illness.

(c)   Two conditions indistinguishable from paranoid schizophrenia have been described – a variety of temporal lobe epilepsy and the amphetamine psychosis.

There are **only two established facts about a possible biochemical basis.** Firstly, patients show impaired response to injections of histamine (the meaning of this is obscure), and secondly, chronic schizophrenics fed with massive doses of methionine (an essential amino acid) rapidly develop an acute psychotic reaction. One view is that an abnormality of the enzyme systems involved in the breakdown of these amines (trans-methylation) probably leads to the local production in the brain of 'psychotoxic' chemicals and serotonin deficiency. (Serotonin, adrenaline and dopamine are naturally occurring amines which act as neurotransmitters in the brain; see p. 149).

Many authorities believe that an abnormality in neuro-transmission is a fundamental factor in the pathology of schizophrenia.

Psychotomimetic drugs which have a similar chemical structure to the neurotransmitters, for example LSD (lysergic acid diethylamide) and mescaline may operate in similar ways. They produce a state not unlike schizophrenia with the important difference that the clouding of consciousness present is suggestive of an organic confusional state.

Neurophysiology

The state of arousal of schizophrenics is odd. Their state of alertness renders them vulnerable to incoming perceptual stimuli and they are very 'resistant' to the emotional demands made by the reception of these stimuli. This is expressed by their flat mood state, indifference and obscureness of language.

The ascending reticular formation, that is, that part of the brain dealing with alerting and arousal, and response to incoming stimuli, is probably involved. In this 'model' of schizophrenia, it is known that:

(a) Amphetamine is an alerting drug increasing the state of arousal and simulating schizophrenia.
(b) Chlorpromazine reduces the sensory input into the ascending reticular formation, reducing arousal and also psychotic symptoms.

It is not understood why many physical illnesses are capable of precipitating schizophrenia and paradoxically allowing many chronic schizophrenics to become more 'accessible' during an acute physical illness.

The signs and symptoms of schizophrenia

There are fundamental groups of signs and symptoms which may occur singly or together in various clinical patterns. The modern tendency is to make a diagnosis of 'schizophrenia' based on the presence of some or all of these symptoms rather than to try and identify or classify the illness in terms of the more rigid subgroups (simple, catatonic, hebephrenic, paranoid, etc.,) which will be discussed later. The groups of symptoms are:

1 Thought disorder.
2 Autistic behaviour.
3 Volitional disorder.
4 Affective (emotional) disorders.
5 Perceptual disorder.
6 Behavioural disorder.
7 Delusions and hallucinations.

1 In thought disorder, the derangement is basically due to three mechanisms:

(a) Condensation (ideas are mixed, having something in common though not necessarily logical).
(b) Displacement (an associated idea instead of the correct one is used).
(c) Symbolization (abstract thoughts are replaced by concrete ones).

The usual logical associations between words and ideas is gradually lost so that speech and thought becomes vague, woolly, confused, illogical, wanders off at a tangent, and is difficult to follow.

This is complicated by **over–inclusive thinking**, where there is an inability in preserving the boundaries of a concept, so that irrelevant thoughts are incorporated into speech.

There is also an inability in differentiating between personal preoccupations and what is going on in the outside world, so that statements about both occur in the same sentence. New words may be invented **(neologisms)**.

The end result of this combination is a meaningless jumble of words and ideas leading to **incoherence** and then **mutism.**

In other cases, there is a sudden block in the train of thought for a fraction of a second followed by a change to discussion of an unrelated topic **(thought blockage)**, or a poverty of thought where the individual does not appear to be thinking much at all.

Disorders of thought content

(a) Primary (or symbolic) delusions are virtually diagnostic of schizophrenia, although they sometimes occur in organic brain disease, e.g. drug induced confusional states and temporal lobe epilepsy. The patient experiences a sudden unshakeable delusional belief that is clearly ridiculous and bears little or no relationship to his usual psychological life, e.g. the sudden conviction that he is God or Jesus. In other circumstances, this type of delusion is the direct symbolic expression of a thought or perception: e.g. hearing a train whistle suddenly indicates that a crowd of people in the railway station is laughing or jeering at the patient. The belief may develop that his thoughts are being broadcast to others or that his thoughts are not his own.

Passivity feelings include the belief that thoughts are being inserted into his mind, or that his behaviour is being controlled by outside forces, e.g. cosmic rays or via television. He may feel **depersonalized** (that his body has changed in some way) or **derealized** (that the environment has subtly altered, is unfamiliar, and there is the feeling that he is losing contact with reality and that his identity is not his own).

(b) Secondary delusions – these are not specific to schizophrenia. However, paranoid delusions are very common; hypochondriacal and grandiose ones less so. Bizarre hypochondriacal delusional ideas sometimes dominate the illness with little or no other evidence of schizophrenia for some years. Typical complaints are, for example, that the nose or face is deformed, that venereal disease is present, or that an organ, such as the heart, is in the wrong place. Secondary delusions may develop in an attempt at explaining a primary delusion, or some of the other bizarre thoughts or symptoms of the illness.

Ideas of reference frequently develop in parallel with paranoid delusions; that is, environmental events assume special meaning – e.g. casual smiles or conversation by strangers indicate some special meaning, perhaps a conspiracy against the patient.

2 Autism is a slow progressive withdrawal from reality. The patient becomes withdrawn, loses interest in his environment, is remote and musing, and preoccupied with fantasy thinking. Eventually, he is dominated by it or by delusional ideas rather than the reality of external life.

3 Volitional disorder is a deterioration in will power, drive and ambition. Apathy may become so profound that self-neglect occurs.

4 Emotional (affective) changes develop insidiously, or suddenly, as episodes of inexplicable depression, elation, ecstasy, giggling or perplexity. The mood change may be related to a delusional belief. The most common change is a **flattening** or blunting of emotion. There is little or no mood display – of feelings such as joy, sorrow or affection to even those closest to the patient. He is offhand and indifferent to people and his illness, and the loss of empathy and rapport has been likened to speaking to the patient through a glass wall. In other cases, the mood is **incongruous**, that is, inappropriate to his thoughts and current situation – so that he smiles when he should feel sad or vice versa.

5 Perceptual changes: illusions (misinterpreting external stimuli), e.g. seeing a face in a flame, and **hallucinations** (a perception in the absence of an external stimulus) are common, especially auditory hallucinations. Hallucinations of taste, touch, sight or smell are less common and raise the possibility of an organic factor being involved, e.g. alcohol or drugs, rather than schizophrenia.

6 Behavioural changes: the withdrawal from reality into phantasy may increase apathy and indifference to the point of complete immobility and stupor (**catatonic stupor**). The reverse may also occur, i.e. **catatonic excitement** – which is purposeless, impulsive, restless, sometimes aggressive behaviour. **Stereotypy of speech and movement** (persistent senseless repetition of words or movements, and the imitation of words and actions (**echopraxia** and **echolalia**) also occur. In other instances, the curious phenomenon of **flexibilitas cerea** is found – the limbs being mouldable into fixed positions for long periods of time, or assumed spontaneously by the patient and having a symbolic meaning. Requests may be disobeyed **(passive negativism)** or the reverse to what he is asked to do done **(active negativism).** Observation of a patient's body movements over 3–4 minutes may reveal various **minor bizarre mannerisms**, e.g. pouting the lips, blinking, grunting, clapping the hands, etc. These are more common in chronic cases. When the above behavioural changes are prominent, the **catatonic** type of schizophrenia is diagnosed.

Physical symptoms are not common in schizophrenia, but a loss of weight and peripheral cyanosis are frequently found in chronic patients, partially due to neglect. **Intellectual changes do not occur**, and orientation, memory and intelligence remain intact, although they may be difficult to test. The patient is invariably **in clear consciousness** although his **insight and judgement are defective**. The typical disorders of thought are sometimes confused with dysphasia or dementia.

Clinical types

The time-honoured division of patients into 'types' rarely fits the individual patient because the symptoms, severity and pattern vary so much with the passage of time. However, because they are so frequently referred to, they require some elaboration.

1 Simple schizophrenia

Develops in adolescence. Apathy, a shallow affect, a lack of drive and initiative and social withdrawal are the predominant features. This is often referred to as disintegration. Delusions and hallucinations are uncommon. Many patients are undiagnosed; many are recluses, vagrants, petty criminals or prostitutes.

2 Catatonic schizophrenia

In this subtype, recurring episodes of excitement or stupor with or without mannerisms (echolalia, echopraxia, stereotyped behaviour, negativism – see under 6 above) are found. Delusions and hallucinations are usually present.

3 Hebephrenic schizophrenia

The onset is in adolescence or the 20s. Emotional changes dominate the illness, e.g. incongruity, fatuousness, or depression. Delusions, hallucinations, thought disorder and personality disintegration slowly develop. The insidious onset sometimes makes differentiation from neurosis difficult.

4 Paranoid schizophrenia

Delusions of persecution are predominant. They may be complex and systematized (i.e. a series of paranoid ideas forming an integrated whole). Hallucinations, usually auditory, are often present. Thought disorder and affective changes are usually inconspicuous. The personality is otherwise quite well integrated. The onset is in the 30s or 40s, and it is the most common subtype of schizophrenia.

5 Schizoaffective psychosis

The dominance of affective features over schizophrenic ones makes it difficult to differentiate from the manic depressive psychosis (see p. 36). The illness may be relapsing, and schizophrenic or affective features dominate the illness at different times. The characteristic feature is that individual episodes respond promptly to treatment with a complete loss of symptoms.

6 Paraphrenia

This is the development of paranoid delusions and hallucinations (chiefly auditory) in a well preserved personality in middle age – 40s and 50s. Other features of schizophrenia are absent.

7 Schizophreniform states

These are acute psychotic reactions which may be genetically distinct from true schizophrenia. They are always precipitated by severe environmental, emotional or physical stress. Typical symptoms include panic, depersonalization, derealization, delusions and hallucinations. The illness clears up rapidly with or without treatment.

8 Schizophreniform states with clouding of consciousness (oneiroid states)

These are rare and may not be genuine members of the schizophrenic family in which **clear consciousness** is nearly always found. They may be, in fact, masked organic confusional states.

9 Pseudoneurotic schizophrenia

Is a term used almost exclusively in the USA to describe certain adolescents who in the UK would be diagnosed as psychoneurotics, with anxiety or depressive symptoms and progressive failure to cope.

10 Chronic (residual) schizophrenia

After many years and repeated episodes, the active symptoms 'burn out' and the residual clinical picture is of a patient who is dull, apathetic, lacking in interest, volition or imagination; invariably deluded, hallucinated and manneristic, sometimes thought disordered, and grossly deficient in insight and judgement.

Diagnosis

Historically, Bleuler's classification of **fundamental symptoms** (thought disorder, affective change, autism and ambivalence of attitudes) and **accessory symptoms** (hallucinations, delusions and all other symptoms) still provides a useful framework of reference for assessing patients.

The diagnostic importance of many symptoms is difficult to assess because clinicians may disagree about the significance. Also, some patients change symptoms rapidly within the course of the same illness. Recent international studies indicate that there is comparatively good agreement that patients who show what have been described as **'first rank' symptoms** by Schneider are definitely to be regarded as suffering from schizophrenia (provided of course that there is no evidence of organic brain disease).

Schneider's first rank symptoms are:

1 Thought insertion (the belief that thoughts are being put into one's mind).

2 Thought withdrawal (the belief that thoughts are being taken out of one's mind).

3 Thought broadcasting (the belief that thoughts become known to others).

4 Passivity feelings (the belief that thoughts and behaviour are being influenced or controlled by others).

5 Hearing hallucinatory voices discussing one's thoughts and behaviour in the third person, or passing a running commentary (e.g. 'he is doing it now').

6 Hearing voices discussing or arguing about oneself.

7 Primary (symbolic) delusions (see p. 36).

A solution to many of these problems has been proposed by **Feighner**, who suggested an **operational definition of schizophrenia** with criteria that do not need to take into account why people become schizophrenic, or whether it is a disease or a defence mechanism. It is merely used as a descriptive label for certain types of abnormal behaviour. His criteria for diagnosis are as follows:

A Both of the following are necessary:

1 A chronic illness with symptoms lasting at least 6 months, without return to the previous level of psychological adjustment.
2 Absence of the symptoms of manic depressive illness.

B At least one of the following must be present:

1 Delusions or hallucinations without significant perplexity or disorientation.
2 A verbal difficulty in communicating due to a lack of logical or understandable speech and thought organization.

C At least three of the following must be present to make a definite diagnosis of schizophrenia; or two for a 'probable' diagnosis:

1 Single status.
2 Poor social and work adjustment prior to the development of symptoms.
3 A family history of schizophrenia.
4 Absence of drug abuse or alcoholism for a year previously.
5 Onset of the illness before the age of 40.

The difficulty with this approach is that it builds the prognosis into the diagnostic criteria discounting the possibility of short lived episodes being 'schizophrenic'.

Differential diagnosis

In the early stages of the illness, when patients still have considerable insight, are alarmed and concerned about their symptoms, and unwilling to discuss them, they are subject to rapid mood changes (depression or anxiety), preoccupation, and sometimes suicidal thoughts. The affective changes may lead to the mistaken label of psychoneurosis. It is not uncommon for patients in this situation to turn to religion, mysticism and various philosophies, or drug taking, in an attempt at explaining the fundamental psychological changes that are insidiously developing. As mentioned previously, many patients in this category would in the USA be labelled 'pseudoneurotic' schizophrenia. Since affective symptoms are so common in schizophrenia, to make a diagnosis of **affective** illness, schizophrenic symptoms must be positively excluded.

The presence of clouding of consciousness usually indicates the presence of an organic disorder or drug intoxication. Some malingerers simulate the symptoms of schizophrenia. A small proportion of severe obsessional psychoneurotics develop bizarre obsessional ideas that become frankly delusional – they may later develop evidence of schizophrenia, but not always.

Prognosis

Doctors and paramedical staff are frequently asked to indicate the long term outlook for an individual patient.

Some of the factors indicating a good prognosis are:

1   Absence of a family history of schizophrenia.
2   A normal personality prior to the illness.
3   A stable home environment.
4   A stable work record.
5   Above average intelligence and social class.
6   Acute onset.
7   Presence of precipitating stresses.
8   Few or no 'first rank' symptoms.
9   Prominent affective symptoms (excitement or depression).
10   Presence of catatonic symptoms.
11   Absence of affective blunting.
12   Initiative and drive retained.
13   Prompt and early treatment.
14   Late onset – over the age of 30–40.

The most important factors are nos. 9, 11 and 13.

Treatment

Modern treatments have dramatically altered the prognosis of schizophrenia. In 1939, two thirds of the number of patients admitted to hospital in the UK with this diagnosis would be there 2 years later. This figure has been reduced to one tenth.

The principles of treatment

1 Patients are initially admitted to a hospital or day hospital for assessment over a period of time. Outpatient treatment is unsatisfactory, especially in more acute cases, because of the patient's uncooperativeness and unpredictability, especially about taking his medication.

2 The signs and symptoms are treated with antipsychotic drugs. Either:

(i) Phenothiazines, e.g. chlorpromazine (Largactil) and thioridazine (Melleril) orally in doses varying from 200–1000 mg daily, depending on the degree of acuteness or excitement. Trifluoperazine (Stelazine) is used in the more inert apathetic patient because of its stimulant properties in doses ranging from 10–50 mg (oral) daily. It is wise to use two or three phenothiazines and get to know them well.

(ii) Butyrophenones, e.g. haloperidol, may be effective where phenothiazines are not; or they may be combined with a phenothiazine. 2 mg i.m. is roughly equal to 75 mg chlorpromazine. As with the phenothiazines, they often produce severe parkinsonian side effects (tremor, restlessness, rigidity, swallowing difficulty and muscle spasm, especially of the lips and tongue) and an antidote must always be at hand (e.g. procyclidine hydrochloride 5–10 mg orally or i.v.).

(iii) Other neuroleptic drugs (see p. 141).

3 ECT is given to patients in whom acute excitement, stupor or a large affective component (depression or elation) is present.

4 Insulin coma, used extensively until the 1950s, has been abandoned.

5 Stereotactic leucotomy is very rarely necessary. It is used in chronic patients who are uncontrollable with drugs and who retain high levels of aggression and tension.

6 Psychotherapy. Analytic type exploration of symptoms (see p. 164) seems to be unhelpful and may help precipitate an acute attack by breaking down the patient's defences. A more supportive type of psychotherapy (see p. 165) is aimed at, designed to help the patient acquire more insight and readjust to his changing lifestyle, family relationships and work possibilities. It is equally important to guide and support the patient's family, whose behaviour may have helped precipitate the illness. These attitudes may be further helped by group psychotherapy.

Nursing care

Is of the utmost importance as it is the nurse who is most in contact with the patient in hospital. It is aimed at helping the patient retain self-esteem and pride, giving him emotional support and encouragement, and acting as a counsellor and possibly a model for behaviour.

Community nurses also assist in clinical assessment and the supervision of drug taking, after discharge from hospital.

Phenothiazine treatment is normally continued for at least a year, and dose reduction is attempted as symptoms improve. Many patients remain on phenothiazines indefinitely.

In unreliable, uncooperative or apathetic patients, **long acting phenothiazines** (fluphenazine decanoate and enanthate) or flupenthixol decanoate, may be given 2–3 weekly i.m. in doses of 25–50 mg instead of oral medication.

Phenothiazines have many side effects (see p. 139) and these easily result in mistakes in diagnosis, e.g. to be mistaken for hysterical symptoms. For this reason, many doctors routinely prescribe antiparkinsonian drugs, e.g. benzhexol (Artane) or orphenadrine (Disipal) whenever moderate to large doses of phenothiazines are prescribed. The obvious alternative is to reduce the dose when extrapyramidal symptoms arise.

The social and work environment in the hospital setting is geared to relieving the patient's anxiety, providing support and encouragement, increasing his social competence and assessing his work skills and potential through occupational therapy.

Many patients, although discharged into the community with residual delusions and hallucinations, are able to live semi-independent lives with some degree of success. This is, of course, helped to a large extent by careful job placement, support and encouragement in the family setting or hostel by social workers, community nurses and general practitioners.

6 Paranoid States

It is 'normal' for most people to develop the exaggerated traits of touchiness, irritability and hypersensitivity from time to time, especially in conditions of psychological stress. In this situation, they are associated with the view that others, or an individual, is selfish or hostile to one. The tendency to ascribe failure, not to our own shortcomings, but to those of others (termed **denial**) is often an associated feature. This is the mechanism of **projection** or self reference responsible for the formation of paranoid ideas or delusions. The subjective bias we have towards our own views further hinders accurate judgement or interpretation of a particular situation.

Psychoneurotics tend to develop this **paranoid tendency** more easily because of their increased vulnerability, self-preoccupation and unresolved conflicts.

Similarly, paranoid behaviour is common in **sociopathic personalities**, the eccentric, social isolate, or the individual pre-occupied with particular religious or political views.

The initial paranoid idea may be based on a simple situation, e.g. a sharp argument over a political view. This later may develop into a paranoid idea relating to a person or topic, which eventually, with time, dominates consciousness and becomes the central theme governing the individual's thoughts and behaviour. It is called an **overvalued idea** when there is a large affective (emotional) component associated, e.g. rage, jealousy, thwarted love.

When the dominating idea becomes fixed and unshakeable, is not open to reason, and is followed by loss of insight, the idea is then clearly a delusion (p. 1) and a **paranoid delusional state** is said to be present. When it exists independently, in an individual whose personality remains otherwise well preserved, it is called a **paranoid psychosis.** It usually develops in early middle age (30s–40s) and may remain for the rest of the patient's life. No other features of psychosis are present.

A paranoid psychosis may be the first development of a secondary illness, for example:

1 Paranoid schizophrenia where other typical affective features, e.g. emotional blunting or flattening, or thought disorder develop.

2 Paraphrenia. A variety of schizophrenia with onset in the 50s or 60s, usually associated with auditory hallucinations and good preservation of personality.

3 An affective psychosis. Either **hypomania or mania** – when a grandiose delusional element is associated, or **depression** with depressive or hypochondriacal delusional ideas.

4 Secondary to organic illness
(a) Transient: e.g. after head injury, epilepsy, drug intoxications (amphetamines, cannabis or LSD) or any confusional state where clouding of consciousness is present. **The amphetamine psychosis** mimics paranoid schizophrenia very closely. Myxoedema, vitamin B_{12} deficiency and Cushing's syndrome are other treatable causes.
(b) Permanent: e.g. associated with dementia, subnormality and chronic alcoholism.

In general, the recognition of a paranoid state or **syndrome is not a diagnosis in itself**, but a diagnostic preliminary, in the same way that the recognition of stupor and depersonalization might be. In this sense, its presence does not have special implications in terms of its permanence, curability, cause, or degree of personality integration.

Deafness, blindness, cultural and social isolation always enhance the possibility of a paranoid state developing. **Psychoanalytically**, paranoid ideas are thought to be the result of unresolved homosexual conflict, or incestuous ideas – perhaps precipitated by an assault on an individual's self-esteem.

Infrequently, an individual or several people living in close relationship in a highly emotionally charged suggestible situation with a grossly paranoid psychotic patient, may 'acquire' or adopt the symptoms and become similarly paranoid and deluded. When one other individual is involved, it is known as **'folie à**

deux'. If two others are involved – **'folie à trois'**. Separation from the psychotic partner often results in loss of the symptoms, but not always.

Treatment

1 The underlying primary illness, e.g. affective illness or schizo-phrenia, must be treated.
2 If the individual's behaviour becomes socially unacceptable or violence is threatened, he should be hospitalized and compulsorily detained if uncooperative.
3 Phenothiazines, e.g. trifluoperazine, relieve tension and reduce the intensity of the paranoid thoughts.
4 Supportive psychotherapy helps build up the patient's confidence. He is taught to ventilate his hostility and eventually face reality. A doctor or nurse may act as confidante and adviser in a 'neutral' way so as not to antagonise the patient.

7 Organic Brain Syndromes

A **syndrome** is a colllection of symptoms and signs that hang together; it may be produced by one cause at one time, and by another cause some other time. For instance when an area of the skin is damaged it first reddens and hurts, then blisters, and finally decomposes to produce an ulcer. This syndrome may be produced by acid on one occasion, by heat on another, or by rubbing on a third occasion. The same is true of those psychological disorders that are caused by disease of the brain (organic brain syndromes). **Delirium,** for instance, may be caused by fever in one patient, and by a reaction to drugs in another. The organic brain syndromes are divided up into:

1   The acute organic brain syndrome.
2   The dysmnestic syndrome.
3   The chronic organic brain syndrome.

The term **acute** is used in its usual medical sense of meaning **short lived** – lasting for days as a rule but sometimes a week or two. Similarly the term **chronic** here means lasting a long time, certainly for months and maybe even permanently. The dysmnestic syndrome is a condition in which **loss of memory** is the main factor: it may be acute (if cured promptly) or chronic (if untreatable).

The acute organic brain syndrome

The acute organic brain syndrome is sometimes referred to as the **acute confusional state** but it is more commonly known simply as 'delirium'. (N.B. It is acceptable to use the term 'delirious' as most people will have some idea what this means. The adjective 'confused' is not so precise, and is used with various meanings by different people.) The main feature of the acute organic brain syndrome is that the patient's **consciousness is diminished**. He is

63

not entirely unconscious of course – it does not make much sense to talk about the psychological state of a comatose patient. He is less **aware** of his surroundings, so that he does not know what time it is, where he is, or who the people are around him. A patient in this state is said to be **disoriented** (or **disorientated**) in time, place and person. These two features of (a) a diminished level of consciousness and (b) disorientation in time, place and person are the central signs of delirium, but a number of other phenomena are seen in many cases. Hallucinations occur and in particular visions are common – e.g. spiders crawling up the wall, or non-existent people Depressive or paranoid **delusions** are seen. The affect may be depressed or elated, and states of anxiety are common. In fact, it seems that **there is no symptom that occurs in the functional mental illnesses that cannot occur in delirium**.

Causes of the acute organic brain syndrome. The most well-known cause of delirium is fever, particularly in childhood. Many drugs will do the same. One particular group is the alkaloid (i.e., naturally occurring type of drug) that is found in the solanaceous plants (e.g., deadly nightshade). This group includes atropine and hyoscine, both of which are used in medicine. There are synthetic drugs which, like these two, give rise to a dry mouth, blurred vision and constipation by inhibiting the action of the parasympathetic nervous system. Some of these compounds are used for treating parkinsonism, and they have been known to cause delirium as a side effect.

Delirium can result from any cause of widespread brain injury. Actual physical trauma will do it, and so will the chemical changes that result from severe major operations, heart failure, or failure of other organs (liver, kidney, lungs). One of the commonest causes of delirium is cerebral arteriosclerosis. In this condition small parts of the brain die off. If the area affected by the necrosis is large, the patient may eventually be left with a paralysed limb, a defect in speech, or some other disability resulting from the loss of function of that part of the brain. During the days immediately following the infarction the patient is liable to suffer delirium, irrespective of the part of the brain affected.

Delirium tremens

Delirium tremens (DTs) is associated in the minds of most of us with alcoholism. After the diminished consciousness and the disorientation, the most striking features of DTs are:

(a) The coarse **tremor** affecting most of the body ('the shakes').
(b) Extreme fear ('the horrors').
(c) Vivid visual hallucinations.

These hallucinations are of 'pink elephants' only in folklore, but animals do often feature in them. Usually, going along with the fearful affective state, these are threatening creatures such as rats or snakes.

It is now known that DTs occurs during the **withdrawal** phase of drug dependence. It has been described not only in alcoholics cut off from their supply but also when patients have come off addictive doses of barbiturates, chloral, paraldehyde, glutethimide (Doriden), methyprylone (Noludar), ethchlorvynol (Arvynol), meprobamate (Miltown, Equanil) and methaqualone (marketed as Melsedin or, in combination with diphenhydramine, as Mandrax).

The dysmnestic syndrome

In this condition the main feature is **loss of memory**. The patient can retain events for only a minute or so. That part of the brain concerned with laying down memory (the limbic system) has stopped functioning properly. Memories of childhood – and adult life up to the onset of the disease – are intact. There is then a gap in recollection until a minute or two previously. In combination with this is **disorientation in time**. If you think about it you will see that you usually need an intact memory to judge what the hour is at present. Ask yourself what the time is now (without looking at your watch) and see how you work it out.

Korsakoff described an organic psychosis in which the above two features were present, and in addition:

(a) Confabulation.
(b) Peripheral neuropathy.

Confabulation is the making up of answers to fill in the gaps in memory. Ask the patient what he had for breakfast and he will give you a fictitious account of sausage and bacon or kidneys, when in fact he had eaten the ordinary hospital scrambled egg. Not all patients with the dysmnestic syndrome will make up stories, though. Just as often they will say 'I don't know' or 'I can't remember'.

Korsakoff's psychosis may result from deficiency of vitamin B_1 (aneurin, thiamin) as, for instance, in alcoholism. Vitamin B_1 is not only required by the neurons in the brain that serve memory, but also by the nerves serving the skin and muscles of the limbs. If these peripheral nerves deteriorate, then numbness, tingling, paraesthesiae and pain (on the sensory side) or weakness and paralysis (on the motor side) may occur with evidence of **peripheral neuropathy**.

To test the patient for the dysmnestic syndrome, give him a fictitious name and address to remember and get him to repeat it two or three times to make sure that he has registered it. Then after ten minutes, ask him to recall it. Most patients with functional mental illnesses recollect it quite well. The patient with the dysmnestic syndrome will be unable to produce more than a few fragments of it, or may not even remember being given the address to remember in the first place (see Appendix 1, p. 193).

Causes of the dysmnestic syndrome include, besides alcoholism, other conditions resulting in vitamin B_1 deficiency (disease of the stomach, gross dietary abnormalities) and vitamin B_{12} deficiency, which is usually, but not always, associated with **pernicious anaemia.** Both B_1 and B_{12} deficiency can give rise to peripheral neuropathy as well. The dysmnestic syndrome can also occur after head injury or encephalitis.

The chronic organic brain syndrome

In dementia, all the intellectual faculties are subject to deterioration, including speech, motor skills, arithmetic, and in the final stages even the ability to wash, dress and feed oneself. These features may not be the most prominent clinically, particularly in the early stages. The patient may present with emotional disturbance, paranoid ideas, personality change or any of the features of the functional mental illnesses. In addition he may show disorientation in time, place and person (as in the acute organic brain syndrome) or difficulty in retaining new information (as in the dysmnestic syndrome). Thus chronic organic brain disease may mimic virtually any other psychiatric disorder.

In the final stages the chronic organic brain syndrome is not difficult to recognize. The patient has lost all his intellectual faculties, and is once again as helpless as a baby. He will lie in bed, with no control over bowel or bladder, unable to care for himself. In the early stages the clinical picture may be misleading, and be dominated by paranoid delusions, depression or hysterical features. Unless the patient is specifically examined for intellectual impairment, the diagnosis may be missed early on.

One sign of dementia to look for is the **impaired ability to learn new information**. It is not true that you 'cannot teach an old dog new tricks' – not unless, that is, the old dog is demented. For instance, if you try to give a demented patient the name and address test that was mentioned earlier in the section on the dysmnestic syndrome, you may find that he is **unable to register the name and address** in the first place. Even after four or five repetitions he is still unable to learn it to repeat it back immediately. The elderly patient without brain disease may have some **difficulty** in learning the address to start with (particularly if he is anxious or depressed) but he will generally be able to repeat most of it at the third attempt.

If a psychologist is trying to detect cerebral impairment, he will give a battery of several tests. Some of these will be **verbal** – e.g. defining the meaning of words, general information – and others will be non-verbal – e.g. completing a missing 'jig-saw' picture, matching designs with coloured blocks. In dementia it tends to be particularly the **non–verbal** tests that are impaired (although in the late stages all suffer).

Clinical forms of chronic organic brain disease

About one in ten of elderly persons can be shown to have some degree of dementia. Postmortem examination shows two types of brain disease in these patients. In **senile dementia** the brain is uniformly shrunken with wide spaces (sulci) between the folds of the cortex and enlarged ventricles – a picture of brain atrophy. Microscopically there are characteristic silver-staining patches (argentophil plaques) and the neurones are distorted by neurofibrillary tangles. In **arteriosclerotic dementia** parts of the brain die off (infarction) to leave shrunken or scarred areas, and the arteries show the underlying disease (usually atherosclerosis).

The typical clinical histories go along with the pathology, so that patients with senile dementia show a progressive deterioration, while arteriosclerotic patients have a series of delirious episodes (at the time of each cerebral infarction) accompanied by a stepwise deterioration. Often the latter patients show a preservation of their usual personalities until quite late in the disease. These typical histories are oversimplified. It is not always possible to tell in life which pathology is present, and at autopsy both diseases are often present together.

Dementia rarely occurs in younger patients. Apart from damage caused by physical injury (e.g. motorcycle accidents) extensive brain damage from specific diseases is uncommon nowadays in developed countries. Psychiatric wards are no longer filled with large numbers of patients suffering from general paralysis of the insane (GPI or brain syphilis) as they were in the last century. In **Huntington's chorea** there is a combination of dementia with the short, jerky irregular movements of chorea. This disease is inherited through a dominant gene, so that on average half of the children of an afflicted adult will develop the disease themselves. In **other presenile dementias** the heredity factor is probably present but not in so marked a degree. In **Alzheimer's disease** there is a general atrophy of the brain, with argentophil plaques and neurofibrillary tangles. In fact the changes are so similar to those that were described above under senile dementia that some authorities would like to include them both under the same name – diagnosing the older patients as 'Alzheimer's disease' too instead of restricting this label for those with the onset under, say, 65 years of age. In another form of presenile dementia, **Pick's disease**, the degeneration mainly affects the tips of the frontal and parietal lobes. One conspicuous clinical difference from Alzheimer's disease is that orientation in space (a function of the parietal lobe) tends to be preserved in Pick's disease so that the patients can still find their way around without difficulty. Often **expressive dysphasia** is a prominent feature of Pick's disease – the patient cannot find the right words with which to express himself. The pathology is quite different to that of Alzheimer's disease.

Investigation of organic brain disease

In the **acute organic brain syndrome** the patient may be suffering from an obvious severe physical illness which is causing his delirium. If it is not obvious his general health should certainly be investigated. It is particularly important to find out if he has been taking drugs, and has suddenly stopped them or lowered the dose (DTs). Often the history of drug taking is denied by the patient, and evidence must be sought from family doctor, relatives and acquaintances.

The commonest culprit is alcohol, and there may be other evidence of alcoholism (cirrhosis, peripheral neuropathy, cardiomyopathy).

With the **dysmnestic syndrome** there may be a history of head injury or encephalitis. Otherwise there may be a clear cause of vitamin B_1 deficiency (alcoholism, carcinoma of the stomach). Serum levels of vitamin B_{12} can be measured nowadays.

The cause of the **chronic organic brain syndrome** is often incurable – senile dementia or arteriosclerotic dementia. Nevertheless even in an elderly patient it is worth considering the possibility of a treatable cause. These include deficiencies of vitamins (as above), endocrine diseases (e.g. hypothyroidism), infections (such as syphilis), benign tumours (meningioma), other space occupying lesions (subdural haematoma), and abnormalities of flow of the cerebrospinal fluid (hydrocephalus).

It may be difficult to tell with some patients if dementia is present at all. For instance, a professor of mathematics can suffer quite a lot of cerebral damage before his arithmetic scores show up as impaired on testing.

Sometimes an electroencephalogram (EEG) may be helpful in revealing brain disease – showing a gross slowing of the brain waves from about 10 cycles per second (hertz) to less than 4 Hz, or showing spiky waves similar to those of epilepsy.

It is sometimes necessary to do special X-rays, either after injecting air (to displace the cerebrospinal fluid and show up the brain in sharp contrast) – 'air encephalography' – or after injecting radio-opaque dyes into the carotid arteries and taking serial pictures as the dye flows through the intra-cranial arteries – carotid 'angiography' or 'arteriography'. These two techniques are potentially unpleasant and carry their own dangers, so one tries to avoid them if sufficient information can be obtained in other ways. A plain skull X-ray is safe, though often uninformative. **Brain scanning** is done by injecting radioactive technetium into a vein and scanning the brain with a geiger counter looking for 'hot spots' that show up tumours. The latest invention is **computer assisted tomography** in which the X-ray machine circles the head taking many shots that are summed up to produce a picture of the contents – all without an excessive dose of X-rays. It is, though expensive, extremely accurate diagnostically. There is no discomfort to the patient. It is often called an **Emiscan,** since the machines are made by the EMI Company.

Treatment of organic brain disease

As with other diseases, the most satisfying treatment is that of the cause. If the cause is untreatable or unknown there is still a lot that can be done in the way of management and symptomatic treatment.

There is much to be said **against** nursing a delirious patient in a darkened room. The patient is already suffering from disorientation, and cutting down on the environmental cues can only make him worse. Even in good light, not to know who it is that is coming into the room, not to know what time of day it is or even (for instance) what meal it is that is being served, can really be a frightening experience. The patient's fears can be allayed if you remind him, as you go in, who you are and then say 'This is your lunch now – it is half past twelve'. It is helpful to have a clock and a calendar prominent, and possibly a radio or television if the patient does not find it too distracting.

On the same set of principles – like giving a crutch to someone who is limping – supportive advice and help of this sort can be given to patients with the dysmnestic syndrome or with early dementia. Those who have difficulty with memory can be helped, if they accept their disability, by getting them to use a notebook and diary. For some people the idea that their brain is affected is itself a painful and distressing notion. In these cases reassurance can be difficult. It may be of help to them to explain that part of their difficulty in thinking may stem from the depression itself, and that they will find it easier to concentrate when they are feeling in better spirits.

In fact some patients with severe depression are in error diagnosed as suffering from organic brain disease.

Drug treatment for the organic brain syndrome

The use of neuroleptic drugs has revolutionized the treatment of the acute organic brain syndrome. In the past there used to be whole wards set aside for delirious patients. Since the introduction of chlorpromazine (Largactil, Thorazine) this has no longer been necessary, and the sight of a patient in delirium is relatively uncommon. Chlorpromazine itself is given in doses of 25 mg to 100 mg, repeated up to 4 hourly. It may be given as tablets, syrup or injection. In some patients it causes a drop in blood pressure or jaundice, so other phenothiazines are often given instead, such as trifluoperazine (Stelazine) or thioridazine (Melleril, Mellaril), which seem to be less likely to cause these two particular complications. Alternatively neuroleptics from other groups are given, e.g. haloperidol – a butyrophenone (see Chapter 17 for further details of neuroleptic drugs).

These drugs are also of value in treating the **chronic organic brain syndrome.** Naturally they will not restore the lost neurons, but they are of help in several ways. They can be given by day to relieve the distress of the patient, or in a larger dose at night to enable him to have a good night's sleep. They act in a quite different way from the sedative and hypnotic group of drugs (e.g. barbiturates, chloral, methaqualone) which intoxicate the patient.

In moderately large doses neuroleptics do not cause the staggering, slurred speech and double vision (ataxia, dysarthria and diplopia) seen with the sedative group. Even with very large doses the patient may sleep but is rousable. The neuroleptics have their effect, then, without unduly suppressing the action of the remaining neurons.

On these drugs the demented patient may change dramatically. No longer is night turned into day. He is calmer, less preoccupied with distracting thoughts, and any bizarre quality in his behaviour tends to disappear. It is easier to communicate with him, in spite of the fact that he still has intellectual deficits. It will be seen that the quality of life may be substantially improved.

Conversely drugs of the **sedative** group should be avoided, since they may make the patient even more disorientated and befuddled. The benzodiazepine group of tranquillizers such as diazeham (Valium), chlordiazepoxide (Librium) and nitrazepam (Mogadon) are variable in effect. Most demented patients can certainly tolerate them in small doses as anxiolytics or sleeping tablets, but they are long acting and may accumulate in the body on regular dosage to cause ataxia.

We have already indicated that in some patients it is difficult to tell how much disability is caused by depression and how much by dementia. Further investigation and observation may clarify the situation but sometimes it is necessary to treat the patient for depression to see what happens. According to some geriatricians there are many elderly patients who are bedridden and incontinent who could be up and about if the depressive element were treated. Usually this means the prescription of tricyclic antidepressant drugs. The elderly patient is poorly able to tolerate side effects (e.g. hypotension) so that low doses are used initially and built up as necessary. In some cases it is necessary to use ECT. Usually this is given when the diagnosis between dementia and depression remains in doubt – it is very gratifying to have the doubt cleared up in a week or two as the (depressed) patient makes an impressive recovery. ECT **can** be given when the diagnosis is not in doubt, i.e. a patient who is known to have both senile dementia **and** a severe depressive illness, if clinical circumstances warrant it.

There is a further group of drugs that are marketed specifically for the chronic organic brain syndrome. They are claimed to increase cerebral efficiency, either by improving the blood flow to the brain, or by a direct action on the metabolism of the neurons. At present they are not universally accepted as being of proven efficacy, though some clinical trials have looked promising. 'Cerebral activators' or 'cerebral vasodilators' in use at present include cyclospasmol (Cyclandelate), dihydroergotoxine mesylate (Hydergine), isoxsuprine (Duvadilan, Defencin, Vasotran), meclofenoxate (Lucidril), naftidrofenyl (Praxilene), fencamfamin (Reactivan) and pyritinol (Encephabol). These names are given for interest – they need not be memorized.

It is not claimed that these drugs can restore nerve cells already dead – the capacity for reproduction has been lost by mature brain neurons. It is hoped that they can improve the function of surviving neurons and if some of these nerve cells are sick to prevent them actually dying off.

This class of drugs is at present undergoing active evaluation, and in future editions of the book it may be possible to be more definite about their place in the treatment of dementia.

Focal organic brain syndromes

So far in this section we have considered the clinical syndromes that result when the brain is affected as a whole. If **one small part** is affected alone the results fall into three categories:

1 Deficits.
2 Release phenomena.
3 Stimulation.

1 *Deficits*

If the part of the brain affected is that part which, for instance, controls the movements of one side of the body, then that side of the body will become weak or paralysed (hemiparesis or hemiplegia).

The part of the brain concerned is in the **posterior** part of the frontal lobe, lying just in front of the central groove or sulcus. The **anterior** part of the frontal lobe governs mental activities such as drive and initiative, self-awareness and self-criticism, and control over one's own behaviour. If this part of the brain is destroyed (e.g. by injury or tumour) or disconnected from the rest of the brain as in the operation of prefrontal leucotomy (see p. 156) the patient becomes apathetic, content to sit and do nothing, and will be prepared to carry out acts that would normally cause him shame, guilt or embarrassment.

Lesions in the occipital and temporal lobes can cause impairment of vision. The nerves from the eyes split up as they pass backwards to end in the visual cortex of the occipital lobes. Destruction of the occipital lobe on the left side means that the patient will be able to see nothing to the right of the midline (with either eye). Destruction of the temporal lobe loses a quarter of the visual field (the upper and opposite quarter).

The most complicated lobe to consider is the parietal lobe. Each half of the brain controls the opposite side of the body, so that in a right handed person the left side of the brain is dominant. Destruction of the parietal lobe on the dominant side of the brain gives rise to

(a) Dyscalculia – difficulty in doing arithmetical calculations.
(b) Difficulty in naming fingers (e.g. which is the middle, ring or index finger).
(c) Disorientation in space – the patient is unable to find his way around the town, formerly familiar environments or even to find his way back to his bed in the ward.

Deficits arising from lesions in the **minor** parietal lobe are less prominent – like the frontal lobe this is a relatively 'silent' area, in that tumours can grow there for a long time before distinctive signs are produced. In severe cases the patient may ignore that side of his body – for instance just dressing the other half.

Dysphasia is difficulty in making sentences or comprehending speech. In **expressive dysphasia** the problem is in uttering words, in **receptive dysphasia** the problem is in making sense out of what you hear. Expressive dysphasia can occur with disease affecting the **front** half of the brain (frontal, anterior temporal or anterior parietal) and receptive dysphasia occurs when the back of the brain is damaged (occipital, posterior parietal or posterior temporal).

2 Release phenomena

When higher centres in the CNS are damaged, control over lower centres is impaired. In the arms and legs reflexes are normally inhibited by the brain; with brain disease any sensation tends to lead to reflex activity ending up with the limb in constant stiffness (spasticity) from muscle overactivity.

Damage to the surface of the brain (cortex) leads to uncontrolled activity of masses of grey matter (basal nuclei or basal ganglia) lying deep inside the brain. This produces the clinical picture of **parkinsonism**, where the patient moves little, with mask-like facial appearance, possibly drooling and shaking, a picture also commonly seen as a temporary sign of high dosage of neuroleptic drugs (see p. 139).

3 Stimulation

A disease may trigger off stimuli in the piece of brain that lies next to it. In the occipital cortex visual hallucinations ensue, in the temporal lobe auditory hallucinations result. Other curious results of temporal lobe disease include (i) tricks of the memory such as the **déjà vu** phenomenon – a conviction that you have seen this particular scene before (although this occurs to many of us occasionally); (ii) surrounding objects looking either very small in **micropsia**, or very large in **macropsia**; (iii) hallucinations of **smell** or of **taste**.

Disease anywhere in the brain may cause **epileptic fits** which will now be considered in detail.

Epilepsy

Grand mal

With a **grand mal** convulsion the patient loses consciousness, holds himself rigid (tonic phase), and then suffers symmetrical and rhythmical jerking movements of the limbs (clonic phase). Some persons are liable to this type of attack throughout their lives, with no cause ever being found (idiopathic epilepsy). Babies may have fits like this when feverish (febrile convulsions), addicts can have them when withdrawing from large doses of barbiturates, alcohol or similar drugs (see p. 65), and they occur in most forms of severe brain disease (under much the same circumstances as delirium may occur).

Petit mal

The patient, typically a child, in an attack of **petit mal** stops eating, talking or whatever he is doing, looks blank for a short space of time, and then carries on as if nothing had happened. Fainting sometimes occurs.

Focal epilepsy

In a focal attack the part of the brain affected triggers off the activity normally under its control, which may be moving some part of the body (e.g. thumb, leg) or it may be producing a sensation such as a taste, smell or memory. This may be the sole evidence of the seizure, but sometimes it is accompanied by loss of consciousness or even by a **grand mal** convulsion.

The relationship of epilepsy to psychiatry

Patients with organic brain disease may present with both psychological and epileptic symptoms, the latter being focal or **grand mal** in type. Alternatively patients who have repeated **grand mal** fits for other reasons may injure their heads during the attacks and end up with organic brain disease.

The textbooks used to describe an **epileptic personality** type (dependent, rigid, religiose) but many experts now think that this description is only applicable to a handful of institutionalized patients. Patients with focal epilepsy in the **temporal lobes** are liable to auditory hallucinations and memory disturbances, and a proportion develop a psychosis with symptoms indistinguishable from those of schizophrenia. Sometimes after a fit a patient will do strange things without remembering his actions subsequently (post-ictal automatism). It is important to be aware of this if a person subject to fits commits a crime – he may not have been aware of his behaviour.

Artificially induced seizures (e.g. ECT, p. 151) are used in the treatment of conditions like depressive illness (see p. 30). We have seen how fits complicate drug addiction. There are many ways then in which epileptic disorders are related to mental illness.

The electroencephalogram (EEG)

Normal electrical brain waves picked up on the EEG are smooth, rounded waves at a rate of about 10 hertz (8 to 13 Hz). Slower waves occur in some otherwise normal subjects, but very slow waves – less than 4 Hz – usually indicate organic brain disease (if the patient is awake).

Epileptic seizures are accompanied by waves that, instead of being smooth and round, are sharp and spiky. They are at irregular intervals in **grand mal** and focal epilepsy, but are rhythmic and accompanied by a slow wave, at 3 Hz, in **petit mal**.

A patient with an area of brain disease, then, may show spikes, or slow waves, or both.

The effects of drugs

Some drugs, including neuroleptics and tricyclic anti-depressants, make epileptic patients slightly more likely to have seizures. Drugs producing the barbiturate–alcohol type of dependence (p. 78) make the patient liable to fits in the withdrawal phase.

Other drugs produce a clinical picture very similar to that of a mental illness. In particular **amphetamine** in high doses (usually in addicts) sometimes produces symptoms that are indistinguishable from those of paranoid schizophrenia. Although the symptoms are the same, the outcome is different. In the case of **amphetamine psychosis** withdrawal of the drug leads to a remission of the psychotic symptoms within a few days, without requiring special treatment by neuroleptic drugs.

The classical picture of **depressive illness** is produced in some patients taking large doses of reserpine – a drug that has been employed as a neuroleptic but is mainly used now in treating hypertension. In this case withdrawal of the drug does not necessarily lead to a remission of the depression, which often has to be treated with ECT or antidepressant drugs. We have seen that delirious states may be produced by the action of some atropine-like drugs, or by the withdrawal of drugs producing the barbiturate–alcohol type of dependence. Otherwise drugs producing florid psychiatric symptoms do not necessarily imitate the naturally occurring mental illnesses. The psychosis of **lysergic acid diethylamide** (LSD), for instance, is not really identical to schizophrenia. Hallucinations occur (predominantly visual), and objects appear to be distorted or seen in a new light. Delusions may occur – the subject sometimes believes that he has superhuman powers. The level of awareness may be diminished, though, and the condition shows some features reminiscent of delirium. LSD is not an addicting drug, but the subject may behave in an impulsive, unpredictable, aggressive or antisocial way under its influence if unsupervised.

Cannabis is a euphoriant drug, producing an (inappropriate) sense of cheerfulness. In large doses it produces excitement and clouding of consciousness. Alcohol reduces anxiety levels. In some people this results in euphoria, but others find it depressing. Contrary to widespread belief it is not a cerebral stimulant, and in large doses causes sleep, coma or even death. However, if the subject is usually inhibited or tightly self-controlled, then the loss of critical judgement produced by alcohol may release uninhibited behaviour, so that the effect certainly looks like stimulation. Further effects of alcohol are dealt with elsewhere (pp. 78 and 130).

Coffee, tea and nicotine probably do act as cerebral stimulants, whether directly or by stimulating the production of hormones such as noradrenaline.

8 Drug Dependence

Dependence on drugs may be either psychological or physical. In psychological dependence the patient feels an intense need to take the drug. The excessive use associated with this **craving** is sometimes called 'habituation'. In physical dependence (or **addiction**) the patient shows (in addition to the above) evidence of a physical adaptation of the body to continued drug use. Evidence of this may be:

(a)   Tolerance to the drug. The addict is able to take far higher doses than normal. Ordinary doses no longer have the desired effect.

(b)   Physical withdrawal syndrome. This is a reaction on stopping the drug which is characteristic of the group of drugs involved. For example the opiate withdrawal syndrome is different from the alcohol withdrawal syndrome.

Dependence on alcohol, barbiturates and related drugs

A good example of a withdrawal syndrome is *delirium tremens* (or DTs). This is similar to other forms of delirium (pp. 63–65) in that consciousness and awareness are impaired, and disorientation in time, place or person occurs. In addition there is often an emotional state of **fear** and visual hallucinations are common. In these visions the patient characteristically sees small frightening animals such as rats and snakes. The characteristic tremor affects most of the body.

   Delirium tremens is usually thought of in connection with alcoholism. In the past it has not always been realized that it is a feature of **withdrawal** of alcohol (or at least a drastic reduction in the regular intake). It is now known that an identical clinical picture occurs on withdrawal of addicting doses of barbiturates and other hypnotic drugs. These include chloral, paraldehyde, meprobamate and also methaqualone (which is a constituent of Mandrax).

Sleep research

Some of the features of drug dependence have been illuminated by recent research using the all night EEG to study sleep. During sleep the EEG tracing shows **spindles** – waxing and waning bursts of waves at 14 Hz. As sleep gets very deep, large **slow waves** occur as well, at a frequency of 1–4 Hz. During the first 60 or 90 minutes of the night we sink deeper and deeper into sleep, and then become lighter again. This cycle repeats itself several times during the night. Every so often a completely different type of sleep occurs, in which there is low muscle tone, irregular respiration and blood pressure, erection of the penis, and rapid eye movements. It is called paradoxical or rapid eye movement (REM) sleep and it makes up about a fifth of the night. If you wake up the subject at this stage he will report dreaming. This means that on average we spend 20% of our sleep dreaming.

Many hypnotic drugs suppress REM sleep, and when they are withdrawn a rebound excess of this stage of sleep occurs, when it may make up 40% of the night. During this rebound the dreams are very vivid and frightening (producing nightmares).

REM rebound in drug dependence

When a barbiturate addict stops his enormous doses of drugs, the REM rebound may reach 100%. What does this mean? On stopping the drug his sleep will be short in duration and intermittent anyway. In other words he will be going in and out of nightmares at bewilderingly frequent intervals. It is small wonder that he will become disorientated and complain of frightening visual hallucinations. It can be seen that our knowledge of REM sleep goes a long way towards explaining the clinical features of DTs.

Recognition of the addict

Observing the occurrence of DTs is one way of eliciting the fact that the patient has become physically dependent on the drug. The development of convulsions is another type of withdrawal syndrome that can occur with exactly the same group of drugs (including alcohol). This seizure takes a form identical to that of the **grand mal** fit of major epilepsy.

Continuous **excessive intake** is not always so easy to detect. It is revealed in alcoholism by the smell on the breath, and sometimes by obvious staggering (ataxia), slurred speech (dysarthria) and double vision (diplopia). The barbiturate addict is not given away by his breath and sometimes successfully disguises the other features. The dysarthria is covered by a slow deliberate speech; the ataxia is not discovered until he is found to be covered in mysterious bruises (presumably from falling over the furniture at home). Double vision is hard to detect unless the patient complains of it; what can be found is nystagmus – jerky movements shown by the eyes when looking to one side.

Otherwise evidence of excessive intake of drugs is indirect. The patient repeatedly claims to have lost the prescription, says that his child has thrown the tablets into the lavatory, or on some other pretext needs more than usual doses to be prescribed. Illegal purchase of the drug is much more difficult to detect. Attempts to inject barbiturates into veins sometimes misfire leading to abscesses, sloughing skin, and scars. Other examples of sedative abuse include glue sniffing and inhalation of anaesthetics.

Other features of alcoholism

Physical dependence constitutes one form of alcoholism. In other alcoholics the intake is sporadic (binges). The patient may find that he can never drink in moderation – he is either abstinent completely or he drinks himself drunk (loss of control). Yet others drink large amounts every day as a matter of course (e.g. in wine producing countries, or in certain occupations) and the seriously high level of intake is not appreciated until they develop a physical complication such as cirrhosis. Some patients drink excessively only while they are in physical pain from a disease, or suffering the distress of a mental illness.

There are other patients in whom the diagnosis of alcoholism is made because drink has ruined their lives from a social point of view. They have lost job after job for turning up to work in an inebriated state, or their marriages have broken up as a result of their drinking and its consequences.

This variety of clinical pictures shows that alcoholism is not a single disease entity.

Opiates and narcotics

There is a characteristic withdrawal syndrome associated with dependence on drugs derived from the opium poppy (e.g. morphine) and powerful pain relieving drugs with similar effects such as heroin, methadone and pethidine (demerol). The syndrome involves loss of fluid from many sites of the body – sweating, diarrhoea, lachrymation, salivation, vomiting, rhinorrhoea – as well as painful muscle spasms and colic. Shivering and gooseflesh occur, and the pupils are dilated (whereas administration of opiates causes constriction of the pupil).

Dependence on morphine and pethidine occurs in professionals who use these substances in their work (doctors, nurses, pharmacists), and in their close relatives. Heroin is mainly obtained illegally. Methadone was used to treat heroin dependence, but now claims its own share of victims.

Amphetamine and other stimulants

Amphetamine is a cerebral stimulant and has been used for keeping air crews awake in wartime. It also suppresses appetite and has been used in the treatment of obesity. This and some other appetite suppressant drugs can lead to considerable tolerance and abuse, but there is not such a clear withdrawal syndrome as there is to opiates or barbiturates. Methylamphetamine is injected intravenously for rapid stimulation. The preparation of drugs for injection by addicts (whether of amphetamines, opiates, barbiturates or other compounds) is often done with poor hygiene – it has even been known for water to be used from the lavatory pan. The consequent hepatitis or septicaemia may be fatal.

Apart from amphetamines the stimulants include methylphenidate (Ritalin), phenmetrazine (Preludin), pemoline (Kethamed, Ronyl) and one of the MAOI antidepressants – tranylcypromine (Parnate). Cocaine causes a similar form of dependence.

Patients on these drugs show dilated pupils, increased activity and restlessness, rapid pulse, loss of weight and sometimes ulcers on the lips (perhaps from abnormal chewing mannerisms). They sometimes develop a paranoid psychosis identical in form to paranoid schizophrenia.

Dependence on other drugs

Dependence on **nicotine** is not associated clinically with a well defined withdrawal syndrome, but some tolerance occurs. Psychological dependence develops rapidly and is extremely difficult to eradicate. As with alcohol, **cannabis** can be used without dependence occurring. It is difficult to reach a balanced conclusion on the abuse potential of this drug because of the extreme attitudes that are taken both for and against it. One possible interpretation of the data is that it has about the same degree of danger as alcohol. Psychotomimetic drugs such as LSD do not usually cause dependence, though there are obvious dangers from their use (see pp. 76–77).

Little is known about the basis of dependence on aspirin (and other mild analgesics) which is rare but definite and which is notorious for subsequent renal damage, particularly from those preparations which also contain phenacetin.

Treatment of drug dependence

Ideally the aim of therapy should be to treat the cause. We should aim at curing the underlying psychological problems that lead the patient to resort to drugs. This is not always possible, either because the psychological problems are obscure or too deep seated. **Psychotherapy** is used for this purpose. Addicts often see themselves as cut off from orthodox society. They may even feel isolated from their psychotherapist if he is seen as an establishment figure. For this reason and others, **group therapy** is sometimes more valuable than individual treatment.

Psychotherapy is fairly ineffective when given to patients that are intoxicated with drugs, and usually abstinence is a condition of treatment. Coming off the drug is a particularly difficult feat for the addict to achieve on his own, so he is often admitted to hospital for this process (referred to as 'drying out'). The drug is gradually withdrawn over a period of a week or two, the patient is helped with his anxieties over this period, and any tendency to fits or DTs is treated medically. The patient may then be discharged for further outpatient treatment, or kept in hospital much longer for milieu therapy (see pp. 164–170).

In the case of heroin dependence an exception is often made to the principle of abstinence, and patients may be given regular doses of heroin or methadone in the hope that at a later stage they will accept complete withdrawal.

For alcoholics motivation may be strengthened by prescribing disulfiram (Antabuse) or citrated calcium carbimide (Abstem). These drugs cause an intense unpleasant reaction to alcohol, and having taken them in the morning, the alcoholic may have his determination not to drink strengthened when he feels tempted later in the day. Unfortunately the reaction produced by alcohol if taken may be dangerous as well as unpleasant. For this and other reasons these drugs are not as helpful in practice as they might seem in theory. Alcoholics may also be helped by former sufferers, and such institutions as Alcoholics Anonymous often prove to be useful (as are similar organizations for other addicts).

In **aversion therapy** attempts are made to condition the patient to associate drinking with unpleasant feelings (such as nausea). This has not been very successful. It may be that behaviour therapy (see pp. 159–163) in other forms will prove more useful in the future.

9 Psychological Development

We shall now look at the process by which the personality is formed, looking in particular at the way in which deviations occur.

First taking a grossly abnormal personality – the psychopath or sociopath – you will recall (p. 4) that such a person is:

1 Antisocial.
2 Impulsive.
3 Guiltless (i.e. lacks the capacity to show remorse).
4 Loveless (i.e. lacks the capacity to give or accept feelings of affection or love).

A core theme underlying these features is **lack of conscience**. How does conscience develop in the normal person? One of the first words that a child learns is 'no', and presumably he learns it from his mother. Let us imagine a small toddler crawling towards the coffee table on which stands a vase of flowers. Suddenly he hears 'No!' thundering out from the woman he had learned to love and trust. He bursts into tears. Love seems to have been withdrawn from him. A few minutes later all is serene once more and he starts off again towards the flowers and the process is repeated. Painfully he learns a lesson. To put it formally, he must **postpone the gratification of his impulses in order to keep his mother's love**. He finds that if he does not do so, he gets a scolding or even a beating. Later, with his friends at school, he might pick up his ball when he is ready to go home. 'You can't go yet – we haven't finished our game' they cry. He finds that he has to put off satisfying his desire to go home if he is to keep the respect of his friends (and perhaps avoid being ostracized or reviled). As an adult he finds that he will avoid certain actions because they are against his own internal standards, and if he **does** impulsively disobey the inner voice he experiences feelings of guilt. This is what is referred to as 'superego' or conscience.

What can go wrong with this process? Firstly, the child may never experience a mother's love for which it is worth postponing any gratification: for instance if mother ignores him. Secondly, mother may be consistently punitive in her behaviour towards him. If he gets punished every hour, on the hour, he may scarcely realize that it is a bad thing to knock over vases of flowers. Thirdly, he may not have a consistent mother figure. If he is passed at frequent intervals from one foster mother to another, then one may punish him for micturating on the floor, but ignore spilled flowers, while another may punish him for spilled flowers but ignore puddles from other sources. It is difficult for him to learn how to please. A child growing up under these circumstances will not go through the normal stages described above.

When he grows up he is likely to be **impulsive** and will suffer **no guilt** if he behaves in an **antisocial** way. This account of conscience development also shows how the early **lack of a loving relationship** can be bound up with these other deficiencies.

This is not the whole story of the factors that lead to psychopathy. Hereditary influences probably play a part, and brain damage from physical injury (during birth or in later life) can distort personality development and behaviour.

Antisocial behaviour itself does not necessarily indicate psychopathy. A man may break the law because he comes from a subculture in which this is accepted as normal behaviour, or because he is psychotic, or even neurotic. Finally he may be driven to it by greed or desperation.

Stages of development

One school of thought (Freudian psychoanalytical) recognizes, amongst others, three early stages of development – the oral, anal and oedipal levels. To many persons the idea is unacceptable that infants derive pleasure (akin to that of adult sex) from oral stimulation in the first year of life, anal stimulation in the second and third years, and genital stimulation in the fourth and fifth years. The concept is more acceptable that during the first year of life development is dominated by **dependency** on the mother, during the second year of life by the **training** process, and during the fourth and fifth years by awareness of tensions between the parents or the other siblings, which may be described as **family rivalry**.

Stage of dependency

At an early age children are clearly very dependent on their mothers, and any threat of parting leads to **separation anxiety**. If separation actually takes place infants rapidly develop depression and apathy.

Maternal deprivation results not only from physical separation but from insufficient affection or consistency of behaviour towards the child. Neurotic behaviour may ensue as a result – e.g. bedwetting, thumbsucking and so on, with a sequel of neurotic behaviour in adolescence or adulthood.

If development is faulty at this stage (e.g. in the first year of life) and a sense of independence does not develop, the person may have enduring problems leading him either to rely excessively on other people (dependent personality) or – though with similar basic problems – to feel obliged to prove continually how self-reliant he is (pseudo-independent personality). To illustrate this, we can see that a person with no difficulties in this area will be able to make his own decisions when this is necessary (truly self-reliant) but when unable to do so (e.g. because he is ill) to accept and trust the decisions made for him by others. In the hospital situation the **dependent personality** may lapse into a passive state in which he allows all decisions to be made for him, and ends up being unable to face the challenge of leaving hospital, with a great danger of becoming a chronic patient. To the **pseudo-independent personality** the big challenge occurs much earlier in hospital if he is put to bed and expected to accept the fact that he is once more in the position of a baby, being fed and even having his toilet needs attended by others. He can be helped to accept this if he is given even small things to do for himself (e.g. complete his own fluid balance chart), thus preserving some of his dignity and self-esteem.

Patients with dependent personalities may come to rely not only on hospitals but on friends and relations, on food, or on drugs. Those who see connections with the specifically **oral** emphasis of the first year of life point out that they may depend in adult life on such activities as eating, drinking, chewing, taking drugs, smoking and talking.

The training stage

The classical example of a hurdle that a child has to pass at this stage is being taught to use the chamber-pot – toilet-training or 'potty-training'. The scene is set when a mother asks 'Do something in the potty for Mummy'. The child pouts and refuses. As soon as he is taken off the pot he releases his faeces. The battle is repeated on later occasions.

A person growing up with unresolved conflicts dating from this stage may show an **obsessional** type of personality. He can be thought of as over-trained – excessively clean, obedient, punctual, and meticulous – he shows character traits of **orderliness**. It is also fairly easy to see how he can end up stubborn and obstinate as well. Some observers have pointed out that such persons are also often very careful with their money, being mean, stingy, or miserly. Others collect things as a hobby. It is not so easy to see why this type of trait should be associated with training. Those who see the importance of toilet training as having a particular significance at this 'anal' stage of development claim that money is 'symbolic faeces'. Lest you think that this is too ridiculous a suggestion, ponder on the terms we use in connection with money. 'Filthy lucre' is possessed by those who are 'stinking rich'. People are 'rolling in it', or, like the colon, are 'loaded'. If you still feel that this is a far-fetched theory, then possibly you can accept that the obsessional personality just likes hanging on to what is his, and resists giving it up.

The stage of family rivalry

The paradigm of family rivalry is the Oedipus complex. According to the Freudian theory at this stage we wish to have sexual relationships with the parent of the opposite sex and to kill off our rival – the parent of the same sex as ourselves. We resolve this conflict by **identifying** with the parent of the same sex. Someone with the **hysterical personality** is said to have unresolved conflicts at this level. Hysterical characters are described as attention-seeking, histrionic (overacting), exaggerating, manipulative, vain, and affectively labile (tears one minute, laughter the next). They show a peculiar combination of being superficially charming or seductive, but underneath being cool and unresponsive.

To explain this further, let us again picture the family scene. This time we imagine a little girl waiting for her father to come home. She hears the latch on the gate and rushes out to greet him. They come in together and he sits there with her on his knee. So far this is an idyllic scene – then mother comes in from the kitchen, hot and tired. 'Go and play upstairs, Jane' she says 'Daddy doesn't want to be bothered just now'. The child easily perceives her mother's coolness and the rivalry for father's attention is clear.

Many of the features described as characteristic of the hysterical personality form part of the normal repertoire of behaviour of a five year old girl, e.g. vanity, affective lability and attention-seeking behaviour. The combination of seductiveness and frigidity, if taken in their literal sexual sense, are certainly to be expected: as for the general sense it is not particularly surprising if little girls are sulky or uncooperative if they do not obtain what they want when they try to be charming. Of course, such manipulative behaviour is normal – a child is likely to try to twist his parents round his little finger rather than use reasoned logical debate.

It is when these behavioural patterns dominate behaviour in the adult that the subject concerned runs into difficulties in his interpersonal relationships, although even then they may be turned to advantage (e.g. the film starlet).

The hysterical personality tends to be diagnosed more often in females, and our illustration has reflected this. Why should this be so? One major factor is probably that of the expectations of our society: it is acceptable for males, when trying to get their way, to thump the table and use overt aggression and forceful measures. It is generally more acceptable for females to use indirect means of persuasion, including tears, drama, charm and other wiles. Perhaps this current pattern will be changed by campaigns for women's liberation.

10 Subnormality (Mental Handicap, Amentia, Mental Deficiency)

All definitions of subnormality use a low intelligence as the most important criterion. It is the only thing that subnormals have in common.

Intelligence is only a rough guide to ability. It indicates the ability of an individual to conduct himself appropriately in the society he lives in, to protect himself from exploitation and common dangers, or to learn social skills adequately.

It is also an estimate of capacity for achievement, before school, at school or as an adult.

It does not take into account the fact that personality factors, motivation (the willingness to organize potential talents in a particular direction), ambition, imagination, perseverence, emotional stability and judgement are almost as important as intelligence in determining the ability to achieve in adult society.

Classification

The old classification of 'idiot', 'imbecile' and 'feeble minded' has been abandoned. The Mental Health Act of 1959 introduced a new terminology.

Subnormality: defined as 'being of a nature or degree which requires, or is susceptible to medical treatment, or other care or training'. (Feeble minded in the old terminology with an IQ below 70.)

Severe subnormality: defined as 'being of such a nature or degree that the patient is incapable of leading an independent life or of guarding himself against serious exploitation'. ('Idiots' and 'imbeciles' in the old terminology with an IQ below 50.)

The World Health Organization (1968) distinction is between profound, severe, moderate and mild mental retardation and the

89

present **educational** terminology separates the educationally subnormal into ESN (severe) and ESN (mild) (see Fig. 3).

Prevalence

In the UK, 2% of the population are subnormal. At least 1 million people have IQs below 70. Three quarters of this group have an IQ between 50 and 70.

The majority function with reasonable adequacy in the community and do not require special care.

Approximately 64 000 subnormal persons in the UK are institutionalized and a further 85 000 supervised by local authorities.

ESN schools cater for 1% of the school population (about 47 000 individuals).

The concept of intelligence

There is no satisfactory definition of 'intelligence'. In general, it is a measure of overall intellectual ability.

Spearman suggested that ability consists of two factors, a general factor (g) and a series of specific factors.

The multiple factor theory suggests:

1 *A general factor (g):* probably inherited, and common to all tests whichever way they are measured.

2 *Specific factors:* which are determined in part by experience, education and environment.

These factors are:

(a) **Numerical.** The ability to use numbers.

(b) **Verbal comprehension.** The ability to understand words and interpret meaning.

(c) **Verbal fluency.** The ability to express ideas in words.

(d) **Spatial.** The ability to visualize shapes and positions.

(e) **Conceptual.** The ability to observe facts, see relationships and draw conclusions.

(f) **Memory.** The ability to remember and reproduce facts.

(g) **Perceptual.** The ability to observe details and interpret them.

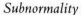

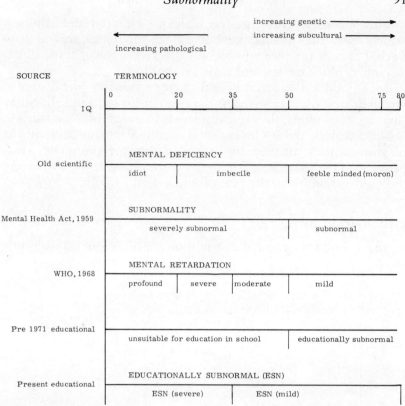

Fig. 3 Terminology of mental subnormality. Adapted from Clarke & Clarke (1975)

There are other abilities, not necessarily measurable with standard tests, e.g. manual dexterity, artistic, musical and creative ability.

Binet–Simon devised simple tests in 1904 for measuring IQ. He used the equation:

$$\frac{\text{Mental age}}{\text{Chronological age}} \times 100 \text{ to give the IQ}$$

It is outmoded and has no meaning in adults.

The Wechsler intelligence scale for children and adults is widely used and measures **verbal**, e.g. (b) and (c) above, and **non-verbal** factors (picture completion and arrangement tests, object assembly, block design and digit symbol tests).

It is a good test in that it has satisfactory **validity** (the degree to which the test measures what it claims to measure), and **reliability** (the degree to which the same results are found at different times).

Nevertheless, the IQ level found need not remain constant. Its measurement is affected by errors of test measurement, inexperience of the tester, test familiarity on retesting, using the wrong test, and variations in the rate of intellectual growth.

Distribution of IQ

Figure 4 shows the normal distribution curve. A low IQ is slightly

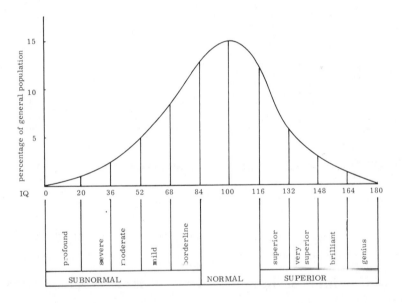

Fig. 4 Intelligence distribution curve

more common than a high IQ, i.e. the curve has a **negative skew** due to the added effect of organic brain disease on the lower side of the curve.

The children of subnormals may be dull but are not necessarily defective. This is due to the tendency for biological regression to the population average so that dull parents tend to have brighter children and intelligent parents to have less intelligent children.

The aetiology of subnormality

1 Heredity

(a) Multifactorial inheritance

In subnormals who represent the lower end of the normal distribution curve of IQ, **multifactorial inheritance** is often present: that is, a number of different genetic factors, which singly would not be significant. Gross physical defects are not normally present. The majority of subnormals fit into this **'idiopathic' group.**

(b) Presence of a single mutant gene

(i)   Dominant inheritance. The affected person has an affected parent and the trait is passed from generation to generation. If an affected person marries a normal individual, 50% of their children are affected.
   Examples are:

   Tuberosclerosis (epiloia)
   Craniostosis (premature closure of cranial sutures)
   Hypertelorism (eyes set widely apart in the skull)

(ii)   Recessive inheritance. The recessive gene must be present in both parents for the disorder to develop in the children. 25% of children are affected. Affected children do not pass on the trait unless it is carried by their marriage partner. The majority are biochemical disorders with a specific biochemical abnormality showing defective synthesis of enzyme necessary for normal metabolism.
   With the exception of phenylketonuria, these metabolic disorders are **very rare.** The following list of metabolic disorders is provided for reference purposes and students whose training requires special knowledge of subnormality:

Amino acid metabolism

e.g. Phenylketonuria
    Homocystinuria
    Maple syrup disease

Fat metabolism

e.g. Tay–Sachs' disease
Nieman Pick disease
Gaucher's disease

Carbohydrate metabolism

e.g. Galactosaemia and glycogen storage disease (Von Gierke's disease)

Disorder copper metabolism

Hepatolenticular degeneration (Kinnear Wilson's disease)

Disordered thyroid metabolism

Cretinism, gargoylism and Hurler's disease

(c)   Disorder of chromosome number or shape

Mongolism (Down's syndrome)
Klinefelter's syndrome: XXY pattern (an extra X or female chromosome)
Turner's syndrome: XO pattern (the male chromosome is absent)

2   Factors operating in utero

Dietary deficiency in pregnancy.
Viral illness in the first trimester of pregnancy, e.g. rubella.
Toxoplasmosis affecting the CNS.
Congenital syphilis.
X-ray irradiation.
Rhesus factor incompatibility (bilirubin encephalopathy).

3   Factors operating at birth

Anoxia – damaging the brain.
Birth trauma.
Prematurity.

4   Environmental deprivation in early childhood

Limits the potential development of any child. For example:
Institutionalization.
Inadequate home circumstances; lack of affection or attention, poverty and overcrowding.

5 Organic defects

For example:

Poor vision
Motor handicap
Emotional disturbance
Epilepsy
Psychotic illness

All inhibit normal intellectual development.
In a recent study, in only a third of 800 cases could a definite cause for subnormality be found. This figure fell to 16% if mongolism was excluded.

The more common syndromes

Mongolism (Down's syndrome) occurs in one in 700 births. There are three different abnormalities:

(i) Trisomy of chromosome 21 is present (i.e. non disjunction). There are three instead of two chromosomes. It is associated with advanced maternal age (usually over 34 years of age).
(ii) Translocation of chromosome 15, a segment of which is found in chromosome 21. It is hereditary and accounts for 20% of mongols. It should be looked for in all **young mothers of mongols** who should be given genetic counselling because of the risk in subsequent pregnancies.
(iii) Mosaicism (very rare) – different cells have different chromosome counts. For example, the skin cells may have the normal 46 and the blood cells 47.

Clinically, mongols have a characteristic appearance. Typically, they have small round skulls, a flat face and a large fissured tongue. Their eyelids are oblique and they have sloping palpebral fissures and epicanthic folds. The fingers are short and stubby and there is a single transverse palmar crease. There is also a large cleft separating the big toe from the others.

Congenital heart disease is frequently present and leukaemia has been shown to occur twenty times more frequently than in the normal population.

The IQ of mongols is usually below 50.

Cretinism may be due to:

A congenital absence of the thyroid, dietary deficiency or a metabolic defect determined by a recessive gene.

A goitre is sometimes present.

The child fails to grow and is slow and lethargic; the skin is coarse and dry, the tongue large and protuberant, and the abdomen distended.

The ligaments around limb joints are lax and the muscles weak.

The voice is frequently hoarse.

Cretins respond to treatment with 15–30 mg thyroid extract daily unless the brain damage has become irreversible.

Phenylketonuria occurs in one in 10–15 000 births. Other aminoacidurias are much rarer.

Phenylalanine accumulates in the serum because this essential amino acid from the food is not converted into tyrosine due to deficiency of the enzyme phenylalanine hydroxylase.

Phenylpyruvic acid is found in the urine. The child is often blond and blue eyed. If untreated, severe retardation, epilepsy, eczema and hyperkinetic behaviour develop.

It is easily diagnosed by special urine and blood tests, which are often done routinely in the first few months of life.

Treatment is a phenylalanine free diet. The prognosis is moderately good in early recognised cases.

Disorders of fat metabolism are all rare. Excessive lipid accumulates in the organs and brain in a progressive way.

Galactosaemia. In this metabolic disorder, galactose is not converted to glucose due to enzyme failure (absence of uridyl transferase). Subnormality with an enlarged liver, jaundice and cataracts is present.

Hydrocephalus may be due to adhesions at the base of the brain after an attack of meningitis or a congenital obstruction to the flow of cerebrospinal fluid. The head enlarges enormously and brain tissue is destroyed.

The obstruction may arrest itself spontaneously or require a surgical shunt operation between the ventricular and vascular systems.

Rubella in the first three months of pregnancy results in deafness, cardiac malformation, microcephaly and subnormality. Termination of the pregnancy is warranted if the mother so wishes.

Congenital syphilis is now very rare. There is a history of repeated miscarriages and characteristic stigmata such as a broad forehead, interstitial keratitis, nasal obstruction and skin rashes.

Clinical assessment

There is no sharp distinction between normality and mental handicap. IQ measurement under the age of five is unreliable. Severe retardation at an early age is unlikely to change. Most retarded children are born to normal parents.

In suspected cases, sampling the amniotic fluid at 12–14 weeks pregnancy detects chromosome abnormalities, some enzyme defects and allows sexing of the unborn child.

In the newborn, a small skull, cerebral palsy, mongolism, asphyxia or convulsions are pointers to subnormality. Most severe subnormals have a **static** brain lesion, and therefore develop in parallel with normal children, but **more slowly.**

A small percentage develop normally, then deteriorate, especially those with metabolic defects.

At school age, the subnormal may present as a behaviour problem, a slow learner, with speech difficulty or as a non-communicating child.

The average IQ in ESN schools is 70.

ESN children fall into two groups: those with cerebral pathology, or those with an unfavourable upbringing.

In the latter group, multiple factors are involved, e.g. dull parents, poor genetic endowment, large families, and emotional neglect.

80% of children in ESN schools make a satisfactory adjustment and are able to work in open employment. 40% of retarded children show behavioural disorder, viz. autism, impulsiveness, irritability, sudden mood changes and overactive hyperkinetic behaviour.

As adults, they may present as drifters or prostitutes with a poor work record, illiterates, or as petty criminals or delinquents.

Management

1. Primary prevention

This includes preventive medicine – e.g. better obstetric care and genetic counselling. Also, improvement of the socio-economic problems or cultural deprivation in a community.

2 Secondary prevention (prompt treatment of detected cases)

This involves early identification of treatable defects such as hydrocephalus, phenylketonuria and cretinism, and the treatment of isolated handicaps that impede development, for example – deafness, blindness, difficulty in reading or in calculating.

3 Tertiary prevention (avoiding unnecessary consequences)

A decision should be made whether home care or institutional-ization is required.

Institutionalization is indicated if severe subnormality is present, especially if the child is emotionally disturbed or has multiple handicaps, perhaps requiring special treatment or education. Other indications are if the child is bedridden and incontinent, or needs constant protection from common dangers. In other instances, the patient's family cannot cope with their presence in the home. Even patients in this group are capable of responding to skilfully offered motivation and simple vocational training.

Home care may be supplemented by **Community care** and attendance at special day centres, schools, assessment units or sheltered workshops. Basic nursing care, through the use of a district nurse or placement in a hospital, involves attempts at retraining a patient in respect of eating habits, dressing, bowel and bladder control and socialization. This requires an infinite amount of patience, tact and support.

Parents, on first learning of a child's mental handicap, react with ambivalent feelings. A wish that the child were dead, guilt because of the wish, anger and projection of their emotions on to doctors and nurses is common. They require a great deal of sympathetic help and support.

11 Child Psychiatry

There are several important differences between child and adult psychiatry.

Children are in a constant state of rapid intellectual and emotional change and development. They are unable to verbalize or express themselves as accurately as adults and they have the capacity to 'act out' their problems and respond to stress with great ease. The 'acting out' in young children is most frequently expressed as feeding, sleeping and eliminating problems.

Children respond to stress in two typical patterns. Firstly, there may be a **regression** to an earlier more infantile form of behaviour and, secondly, the **normal responses in development may persist** for long periods of time, e.g. soiling and wetting in infancy, temper tantrums in 2–4 year olds, separation anxiety in children under 5, and preschool phobias in older children.

Symptoms should always be evaluated in respect of their effects on the total function and development of the child. This includes motor and language development, personal and social behaviour, and the way in which the child adapts to its environment as a whole.

The family, parents and siblings must always be intimately involved in the diagnosis and treatment of the child. Therefore, a detailed and adequate history is essential. This must include details of birth, the development of milestones, the presence of congenital abnormalities, inherited illness, birth injury and subnormality.

The social and emotional relationships in the home and at school are particularly important, so as to provide an 'in depth' picture of the total background to the child's problems.

An independent history from the parents and siblings is taken, if necessary.

The mother's attitudes and attentiveness to the child, and the father's role in the family, must always be enquired into. Either or both parents may show evidence of persistent unreasonableness towards the child via their excessive demands, over-strictness, irritability, cruelty, over-protectiveness or anxiety.

The birth order, evidence of sibling rivalry, and evidence of tensions in the family due to marital stress, divorce or separation, or formal psychological illness in other members of the family are also evaluated.

The ethnic, racial and religious, and socioeconomic background are other factors to be taken into consideration.

In adolescents, more attention is paid to the adequate development of relationships with parents, siblings and peers, the self image, sexual status and the possibilities of latent homosexuality and masturbatory guilt. Discrepancies between the intellectual level of the child or adolescent and the expectations of family and school need to be assessed.

It must be realized that the presenting symptoms may be the tip of an iceberg and indicate the first presentation of more serious family problems, either specific personal or family crisis.

In general, psychiatric abnormality must not be inferred on the basis of the development of a single new item of behaviour.

The **interviewing** of a child needs to be tactfully and sensitively handled. A detailed physical examination, especially of the central nervous system, intellectual assessment and psychological testing, are essential parts of the total assessment. Play therapy may be required if the child is non-verbal. The home and school may be visited by a social worker in order to obtain a broad independent view of the background.

Problems of infancy and the pre-school years

As with most behavioural disorders in childhood, these problems are the reflection of rejection by parents, lack of affection, insecurity, fear, depression, unresolved conflicts with consequent anxiety, and displaced aggression.

The maladaptive behaviour that follows results from inefficient use of psychological defence mechanisms (see Chapter 9).

The majority of the disorders are transient and respond to appropriate relief of the underlying causes. **The more common disorders are:**

1   Thumb sucking.
2   Rocking and head banging.
3   Excessive masturbation.

4 Food refusal and pica (the ingestion of non-food materials).
5 Temper tantrums.
6 Fidgetiness and hyperkinetic activity (restless, overactive, distractible behaviour). The latter may result from brain damage, post encephalitis, or be associated with epilepsy or mental retardation.
7 Sleep difficulties – insomnia, night terrors and sleep-walking.
8 Speech disorders – short periods of stammering are common in 4% of children between the ages of two and six. There is often a family history. Stammering itself is not a sign of psychiatric disorder. It is always increased by anxiety and may secondarily result in neurotic behaviour in the insecure, ashamed, self-conscious child. It is generally outgrown. Some cases require intensive speech therapy or behaviour therapy.
9 Disorders of toilet training
(a) Encopresis (faecal soiling after the age of 3) usually indicates poor training. In encopretic children, painful anal fissures and constipation are commonly found. Many are dull intellectually and they may be enuretic. In older children, obsessional behaviour and conflict with the mother are often present. The child is frequently very disturbed and anxious.
(b) Faecal smearing in older children is evidence of anxiety or mental retardation.

Enuresis

Enuresis is one of the most common symptoms found in young children. Bladder control is normally achieved by the age of 5, more rapidly in girls than in boys. There are two types of enuresis:

In **primary enuresis** the child is enuretic from birth. Failure of adequate training, especially in the mentally retarded, is the commonest cause. Organic causes need to be excluded, for example, genitourinary infections and malformations, spina bifida, epilepsy and diabetes.

In **secondary enuresis** there is a period of normal bladder control followed by bedwetting. It is most likely to be a regressive symptom, related to emotional stress. Other symptoms may be associated.

In older children, secondary psychological problems, anxiety and guilt may develop as a **result** of the enuresis.

Abnormally deep sleep is sometimes associated and responds to treatment with 5–10 mg amphetamine at night.

In most cases, treatment with a tricyclic antidepressant is very helpful.

More resistant cases require deconditioning using an electrical alarm circuit wired to a pad. Urination completes the circuit by wetting the pad and a bell rings, waking the child. Eventually this occurs before full urination is completed.

Neurotic disorders

These are more common in the school-going child or adolescent. Although they conform to the adult pattern of neuroses – anxiety states, obsessional compulsive behaviour, phobic disorders, conversion and dissociative states, and reactive (neurotic) depression, they are more changeable and less clearly differentiated.

The majority of neurotic behaviour in children is no more than the temporary exaggeration of a normal developmental trend.

Depression, as it presents in adults, is uncommon, but reactive depression does occur. It is more common for depression to present in a masked form as obesity and compulsive overeating, hypochondriasis, accident proneness or truancy.

Psychosomatic symptoms may similarly indicate depression, or be related to anxiety and tension states. Common psychosomatic symptoms are persistent headaches, diarrhoea, constipation, stomach and limb pains, asthma and eczema, and facial or body tics.

School refusal or school phobia in adolescents (10–14 years olds) may be associated with other neurotic symptoms such as shyness, fears, and separation (from the mother) anxiety. The mother may be over-protective and anxious.

Personality disorders

These disorders are more common after the age of 9 or 10. The pattern of behaviour is determined by the personality type, e.g. paranoid, obsessional, hysterical or schizoid.

Multiple neurotic symptoms are found interwoven with delinquent behaviour, truancy, aggressiveness and resentfulness of authority. Evidence of insecurity and anxiety is usually present.

As in neurotic disorders, emotional deprivation and consistent neglect or cruelty by parental figures are contributory.

A percentage of patients have an organic basis to their illness, for example after an encephalitic illness, in epilepsy, brain damage and mental retardation.

The prognosis for essentially normal children committing isolated antisocial acts is good.

Significant numbers (30–40%) of children with personality disorders extend their disorder into adulthood. This includes the group of adolescents with states of 'emotional turmoil' and prolonged identity crisis.

Psychoses in children

The diagnosis of a psychosis in a child must be preceded by the exclusion of several other conditions that mimic psychoses, e.g. deafness, aphasia, mental subnormality, brain damage and a severe neurotic or personality disorder.

There are two common psychoses:

1 Autism.
2 A schizophrenia-like psychosis.

1 Autism

The syndrome of autism was first described by Kanner in 1943. It was though to be a variant of childhood schizophrenia. This view is no longer tenable.

Autism occurs in 2–4 per 10 000 children and is more common in males in the ratio of 4:1. The parents of autistic children tend to be above average in intelligence.

The symptoms may develop insidiously from birth or present at the age of 2 or 3.

The autistic child is cold, aloof and lacks warmth and interest. He is unable to relate in the ordinary way to people – including parents and siblings, or to his environment as a whole. The child has an obsessive need to maintain the 'sameness' of his environment, and any change results in attacks of irritability, rage and panic.

They are fascinated with inanimate objects and indulge in aimless repetitive mannerisms, e.g. rocking, chewing and spinning of the body.

There is a failure to use language as a means of communication, and some afflicted children have no speech at all. Others use speech abnormally, talk to themselves, repeat the spoken word or phrase (echolalia) or show pronominal reversal (e.g. use 'you' for 'I').

Careful testing shows that most autistic children have in fact good intellectual potential and are able to develop reasonably high levels in motor skills.

The severity of the illness varies from total autism with aimless repetitive behaviour to the odd eccentric aloof schoolboy.

The prognosis is poor and only 14% make a satisfactory school and social adjustment. 60% have a poor outcome and need long term hospital care.

Autistic children require a great deal of encouragement and attention. They are best placed in special schools. Attempts at treatment are made by the positive reinforcement of desirable behaviour.

The aetiology remains in doubt. A biochemical basis or a perceptual abnormality have been suggested. Parents often have schizoid traits and a hereditary factor may be involved. In most cases it is thought that the child's failure to master separation anxiety from the mother is important.

Secondary autism frequently develops in the presence of (associated with) brain damage or mental subnormality.

2   A schizophrenic type psychosis

This has been described developing in children of 5–6 years or older. It may present as mental retardation or as a neurotic illness. The child is typically withdrawn, remote, irritable and subject to temper tantrums. Paranoid features and excessive preoccupation with fantasy life may be present, and also evidence of loosening of associations and thought processes along the lines of typical schizophrenic thought disorder. As a consequence, intellectual development is seriously hindered. Bizarre stereotyped movement and identification with inanimate objects may be present. Remissions in affected children often occur at puberty. Adult types of schizophrenia are seldom seen in children.

Organic brain syndromes

An acute brain syndrome characterized by rapid delirium, clouding of consciousness and hyperpyrexia are common features of many childhood illnesses.

The illness is invariably followed by a dramatic reversal, without sequelae, to normal.

In adolescence an acute confusional state secondary to emotional stress sometimes develops. Its onset is abrupt. Acute anxiety, depression, confusion, depersonalization and disorientation are found.

Improvement follows rapidly when the provoking causes are removed.

Chronic brain syndromes usually follow brain damage at birth or later. Neurological deficit, speech disorders, and cognitive loss (in memory, judgement, comprehension and learning ability) are associated with some degree of intellectual retardation.

If partial or complete recovery occurs, long term sequelae may be present, such as epilepsy and personality changes along the lines of aggressiveness, irritability and antisocial behaviour. Hyperkinetic behaviour is commonly associated.

Specific reading disability (dyslexia) occurs in 5–10% of school children at all levels of intelligence. Their inability in dealing with letters and words as symbols is probably due to a basic fault in cerebral organization and dominance. Secondary neurotic developments are common.

They require remedial reading and phonetic retraining.

Treatment of childhood disorders

The modern approach is to have a treatment team in either a hospital outpatient clinic or child guidance clinic. The team consists of a child psychiatrist who has overall clinical responsibility, a psychologist who is responsible for the assessment of intellectual and educational aspects and some forms of treatment, and a social worker who helps with the treatment of the parents, explores social factors, and helps with the better integration of the family into the community. Some clinics have lay or medical psychotherapists.

A sensible formulation of the diagnosis and possible lines of treatment depend on correct appraisal and assessment of the patient in the context of his life history, background, family and environment.

Explanation and advice to the parents – the most influential factors in the child's environment – is always a part of treatment.

Insight-orientated psychotherapy may be required, either individual, group, psychodrama or play therapy.

The social environment may need changing. The child may have to be moved to a hostel, foster parents or to a hospital.

Drugs and ECT play similar roles as with adults, but are required less often.

Nursing care provides a useful supportive role and mother substitution.

Many child psychiatrists use a behavioural diagnostic approach and treatment is designed using an appropriate behaviour therapy technique. This is based on the view that many childhood psychological illnesses result from a breakdown or maladaptation of learning principles. The treatment aims at deconditioning the child to the maladaptive behaviour.

Although spontaneous recovery is common in the psycho-neuroses, children with psychoses rarely recover and the presence of a personality disorder implies an extended disorder in time.

In general, the kind of problems present in childhood portend in type adult psychiatric illness, but there is no way of knowing who will or will not develop psychological illness as an adult.

12 Psychosexual Disorders

Normal sexual behaviour

Patterns of morality, social codes and customs vary so much in different countries, and from culture to culture, as well as changing even over short periods of time, that it is difficult to define what is normal or abnormal in sexual behaviour. The term abnormal consequently tends to mean 'unusual' rather than 'pathological'.

Most frequently, it is the legal as well as the social system in a particular country which determines what is acceptable sexual behaviour.

By 'normal' sexual behaviour is usually meant 'any activity which in heterosexual relationships leads to intercourse and orgasm'.

Masturbation is regarded as being normal (usual) practice in children and adolescents, and in adults deprived of a sexual partner. It tends to be excessive in maladjusted personalities, the mentally subnormal and in schizophrenics.

Psychiatrists have, in the main, discarded the term 'sexual perversion' and have substituted 'sexual deviation' or 'minority sexual practice' as more acceptable alternatives in line with the changes in attitude of society over the last few decades.

The amount of sexual deviance present in particular societies or cultures is difficult to ascertain. The majority of people who indulge in deviant behaviour do not seek help from psychiatrists and are likely to be reticent about revealing their sexual behaviour because of guilt feelings, shame, shyness or social taboos.

Recent studies, however, do seem to indicate that sexual problems, as well as deviance, are extremely common, especially in Western type cultures, and that the commonest problems are various types and degrees of **impotence** in men and **frigidity** in women.

The differences between the sexes, apart from their anatomically distinct genitalia, are to a large extent determined by psychological factors exerting their influence in childhood and adolescence. They

107

include parental influences, the nursery and the school, and environmental conditioning through the media, religion, and interpersonal relationships.

The male is trained or conditioned towards assertiveness, aggression and 'masculine' sports and interests, and the role of being a provider of protectiveness and material requirements, whereas the female is trained to a more submissive role – which is primarily maternal and domestic.

In the last few decades, women have become more assertive and have, with some degree of success, attempted to liberate themselves from this assigned role and what is regarded as male chauvinism.

It is of interest that children brought up from infancy as the opposite sex invariably behave and think as that sex. That is, they have a subjective sense of sexual identity or **gender role.**

Aetiology

The causes of sexual deviation are not clearly understood. **Heredity** does not seem to play an important role, except perhaps in a very small proportion of homosexuals. **Psychoanalytic** explanations provide a theoretical framework upon which treatment is frequently based.

In psychoanalytic theory, children are thought to pass through several developmental phases (see also p. 85):

(a) The oral phase which is sexually pleasurable because of sucking and biting.

(b) The anal phase where pleasure is associated with the retention and expulsion of faeces.

(c) The phallic phase where pleasure is derived from the individual's own body and genitalia. This is the basis of

(d) Adult sexuality, where the interest is directed towards the opposite sex.

If psychosexual development is **inhibited or fixated,** that is, there is a failure to develop beyond one of these earlier phases, then adult sexuality assumes some of the features associated with that infantile phase. For example, fixation at the oral phase is associated with biting or sadistic behaviour, and fixation at the anal phase is associated with obsessional and fetishistic behaviour.

In the **oedipal** (or phallic) phase of development (where there is close identification with a parent of the opposite sex), fixation results in a failure of identification, in later life, with a parent of the same sex. As a result, incestuous guilt feelings develop with doubt and concern about one's sexuality.

Over-protective domineering mothers or weak, ineffectual or violent aggressive fathers are supposed to be related to this failure of identification. Although the influence of **heredity** in determining these fixations is not clear, **environmental conditioning** is probably of considerable relevance.

For example, parental attitudes condition a child to behave in particular ways. Sexual guilt is easily acquired if the child feels unable to conform or expresses differing views or hides his sexual feelings.

Similarly, sexual assaults in childhood, or incestuous relationships or fantasies produce guilt feelings which might be symbolically displaced in one or other variety of adult sexual deviance.

In general, the presence of sexual guilt or fear (which may be of real or imagined terrors) is invariably associated with adult sexual problems or deviance.

Psychosexual disorders may be subdivided into:

1   Sexual dysfunction, e.g. **impotence in the male** and **frigidity in the female.** The varieties of these two conditions are by far the commonest problems.

2   Sexual deviations

The more common deviations are:

(a)   Homosexuality and lesbianism
(b)   Transvestism and transexualism
(c)   Exhibitionism
(d)   Fetishism
(e)   Sadomasochism
(f)   Voyeurism

and other conditions which might be far commoner than formerly supposed, e.g. obscene letter writers and phone callers.

In this scheme, sexual deviation may be defined as 'any sexual activity or fantasy, other than sexual intercourse with a willing partner, which leads to orgasm, and which is usually repeated over an extended period of time'.

Impotence in the male

Impotence is 'the inability to achieve or maintain erection to the point where coitus is completed with orgasm'. It may present in various ways: either as total or partial lack of libido (sexual drive), inability to have an erection even if libido is present, inability in maintaining erection, premature ejaculation, inability to ejaculate, or ejaculation without orgasm.

The majority of men ejaculate within 2 minutes, whereas women take three or four times longer to achieve orgasm. In premature ejaculation, ejaculation occurs before or shortly after vaginal penetration.

Two types of impotence are described

1   Primary impotence which is present from the first attempts at intercourse. It is most frequently associated with individuals who are anxious and insecure, lack assertiveness or fear aggression on the part of the female. Latent homosexuality, castration fantasies, and unresolved guilt feelings concerning childhood sexuality are all thought to play a part in its development.

Other considerations that need to be enquired about are fears of venereal disease or pregnancy, and undue respect for the female partner (performance with a prostitute may be perfectly adequate).

The impotence may be temporary, variable, or permanent. The subsequent humiliation and anticipation of failure produces a conditioned cycle of anxiety, so that the anxiety is constantly reinforced and further increased by the inevitable tension of the female partner. The end result is a progressive increase in anxiety and diminution in performance.

2   Secondary or late onset impotence occurs after a period of adequate sexual adjustment. It is more common in middle life – in the forties and fifties.

It is most frequently due to boredom with the female partner, or personality clashes in advancing age due to changing emotional needs, interests and attitudes. Psychological illness, e.g. depression or anxiety, frequently precipitates the development of secondary impotence. In other cases it may be associated with organic disease, e.g. peripheral neuropathy as in diabetes, alcoholism, multiple sclerosis or endocrine disorders. Antihypertensive and anti-depressant drugs and steroids are other potent precipitants.

At the age of 70, about 50% of men are still potent. Biologically, potency begins to decline slowly from the middle 20s and more rapidly after 55–60.

Frigidity in the female

Frigidity is 'the inability to become sexually aroused or to achieve orgasm' in heterosexual relationships.

It varies from a total lack of desire to desire without achieving orgasm, or orgasms only achieved by external stimulation of the female genitalia. The latter category is in fact a biological norm, and the large numbers of women presenting with this complaint should be made aware that their anxiety is to a large extent culturally determined.

In other instances, dyspareunia (painful intercourse) is associated or vaginismus (painful spasm of the vaginal barrel before or after penetration).

As in the male, it may be primary or secondary.

1 In primary frigidity, which exists from first attempts at intercourse, the individual is usually immature, vulnerable, and has hysterical traits, or other evidence of personality disorder.

Latent lesbianism (with penis envy and rejection of the female role) or primitive fears of damage by the penis, fears of pregnancy, or guilt concerning the sex act, are other related causes.

2 Secondary frigidity occurs after a period of normal sexual activity.

As in the male, boredom, sexual disinterest and disenchantment, or personality clashes, are the commonest causes. Excessive demands by the male are frequent complaints.

Organic causes and depressive illness need to be excluded, as well as local lesions causing pain or irritation.

Frigidity sometimes develops too because of the male partner's inefficient technique or premature ejaculation.

There is no evidence that libido diminishes significantly immediately after the menopause, but as in the male, the libido slowly wanes with advancing age.

The treatment of impotence and frigidity

Most patients never see a psychiatrist, despite the considerable anguish and marital tension that is present.

Organic causes, and anxiety or depression must be appropriately treated.

In the majority of cases, the causes are primarily psychological and the symptoms are a direct index of underlying personality problems, fears or conflicts. Accordingly, a full and detailed history from both partners is always necessary as a prelude to psychotherapy. Joint interviews may be necessary, and even ostensibly simple problems such as jealousy, competitiveness and failure to make compromises in a relationship explored. Environmental stresses such as job dissatisfaction, loneliness or financial stress may be important.

A detailed physical examination is always made.

Many people have surprisingly naïve, limited or ignorant ideas concerning expectations and sexual technique. Simple ventilation of these may in itself prove to be therapeutic.

If the problem is a recurring one with different sexual partners, the patient's personality, life style, and emotional adjustment need more careful and detailed exploration. Joint marital therapy or anxiety relieving behavioural reconditioning techniques, as described by Masters and Johnson, are often very helpful.

Hypersexuality

This is the need or desire for an excessive amount of sexual intercourse. It is not possible to define what is 'abnormal' in this sense, but psychiatrists may be asked to see people whose conscious thoughts are dominated by sexual preoccupation to the point where they interfere with the individual's life style, work, and relationships, despite their excessive indulgence in sexual activity.

In these instances, the sexual act rarely provides emotional satisfaction and the condition is a reflection of underlying psychological problems or illness (e.g. hypomania, some schizophrenia, organic brain disease or personality disorder). In the last, hypersexuality usually indicates a basic sense of sexual insecurity or inferiority and the need to repeatedly and compulsively 'prove' sexual adequacy and desirableness.

Psychodynamically, unresolved oedipal conflicts are thought to be present, that is, attempts are made – in vain – to find a maternal or paternal figure who can satisfy their idealized expectations.

Organic causes include damage or degeneration in the hypothalamic area of the brain, and temporal lobe epilepsy.

The premenstrual phase in women, amphetamines, opiates and androgens, also increase the libido.

Many cases are referred to psychiatrists through the courts – where sexual assault, rape or intimidation have occurred.

Homosexuality

Homosexuality is defined as a 'sexual interest or relationship with people of the same sex'. In the female it is also referred to as **lesbianism.**

Most homosexuals are on a continuum varying at one extreme from complete heterosexuality to complete homosexuality at the other, with some people in the middle having sexual interest in both sexes.

Kinsey's figures indicate that:

In males, approximately	10% are exclusively homosexual
	37% show some evidence of homosexuality
In females,	6% are lesbian
	28% show some evidence of lesbianism

The causes of homosexuality are obscure. Although chromosome studies are normal, it is thought that a genetic factor may be involved. It is not related to known endocrine disease.

The **gender role** is of some significance: that is, whether the child was brought up as a male or female, and its relationships with the parents. The acquisition of sexually orientated behaviour in early childhood may be in part by imitation or modelling.

Some analysts believe that male homosexuals, as a result of early painful emotional experiences, are prone to see women as sharp and critical, and therefore they are liable to feel intense anxiety when in intimate physical proximity to a woman or in social situations.

A more recent view is that heterosexuality is the biological norm and that homosexuality results from fears concerning heterosexuality: that is, that all homosexuals are latent heterosexuals.

Most homosexuals are both active and passive in their habits. Because less stigma is attached to lesbianism in most societies, such women are infrequently seen by psychiatrists. When they do, they present with far less anxiety and conflict than males, and are less liable to exposure, ridicule and blackmail.

Exclusive lesbianism is rare and lesbian women frequently have children. As with male homosexuality, the causes are obscure. Loneliness, isolation in a female society (school or prison), fear of rejection by a male, or childhood sexual trauma in association with a male figure are all relevant.

Homosexuality and lesbianism are so common as to be regarded as a **normal variation of sexual behaviour** and **not** as pathological behaviour.

Homosexuals only require treatment if they are unable to accept the implications, or come to terms with their sexuality in the setting of the society they live in and its strictures: e.g. if they are unable to cope with shame, guilt or inferiority feelings, or where there is an associated personality disorder and that the individual is unable to form meaningful or lasting relationships. Homosexuals who are unhappy at being so are helped to understand and deal with their conflicts.

Certain homosexuals who wish to become heterosexual are often treated with behaviour therapy (which regards homosexuality as a learned pattern of sexual behaviour). Attempts are made at modifying or diminishing the homosexual drive by using aversion or avoidance therapy, using electrical or chemical stimuli to produce disgust, pain or nausea.

Sadomasochism

Sadomasochism is, to a minor degree, present in most individuals, if only in their social behaviour or in the form of occasional sadistic or masochistic fantasies.

In the strict sense, **sadism** means the achievement of sexual pleasure or orgasm by the infliction of pain or cruelty upon another individual (male or female) or upon an animal.

It ranges from 'acceptable' minor sexually sadistic acts such as biting and scratching during sexual relations to severe whipping and beating, rape or even murder.

In gross forms it is predominantly found in males.

Socially sadistic behaviour may be evidence of repressed sexual sadism.

Masochism

This usually co-exists with sadism. It involves the infliction of pain or humiliation upon the self in a deliberate way in order to achieve sexual satisfaction. It is thought to be one way aggressiveness is displaced or 'turned inwards' on the self – the need for punishment being satisfied because of incestuous sexual desires towards one or other parent in childhood.

Because so much social behaviour is consciously and unconsciously sadomasochistic, it is found to be an important element in many personality disorders.

Psychotherapy is of limited usefulness. Many patients are treated with some success using behaviour therapy (aversion deconditioning techniques).

Transvestism

This is the term used to describe the wearing of clothes of the opposite sex in order to achieve sexual excitement. It may be the only way in which an individual is able to achieve orgasm. It is more common in males, and is present in most cultures. It is a form of fetishism (see p. 116).

Many transvestites lead reasonably stable and contented married lives, reserving their cross dressing for periods of sexual isolation, loneliness, emotional stress or depression. On the other hand, it may become a regular habit accompanied by masturbatory fantasies. These are often of identification with a mother or sister or involve an incestuous relationship with one or the other. An identification with a female figure (for the male) in childhood is thought to result from the inability in forming a normal identification with his father.

Repressed homosexuality may also be associated.

Transvestites infrequently seek psychiatric help. Many are seen after a court referral – frequently on charges of stealing women's underclothes or clothing.

Psychotherapy may help their adjustment but seldom alters their habit.

Behaviour therapy using electrical aversion methods is often effective in reducing the frequency of cross dressing in individuals in whom it has become a social problem.

Transexualism

Is the term applied to a small group of persons who have the firm conviction that they belong to the opposite sex despite their anatomical normality.

They do not respond to formal treatment of any kind, remain unhappy, and are dominated by the desire to change their anatomical sex by plastic surgery.

Many such individuals do end up by having operations, yet seem unable, nevertheless, to make a satisfactory psychological adjustment.

Their **cross gender** identification begins in early childhood. In some instances, the individual is found to have been brought up and dressed as belonging to the opposite sex. In other instances, the transexualism is evidence of a schizophrenic delusion.

In a further small minority, pseudohermaphroditism is present and discovered at puberty, when the child, brought up as a female because of having rudimentary male genitalia, develops more obvious evidence of being a male (enlarged penis, testicles, beard growth).

Fetishism

In this deviation, sexual arousal or orgasm is achieved in relationship to seeing, touching or wearing inanimate objects, e.g. rubber garments, leatherware, women's underwear, shoes, etc.

The fetishistic object may be part of the anatomy of the opposite sex partner – viz. hair, penis, breasts or buttocks. Compulsive theft of fetishistic objects frequently provides the sexual excitement.

Most fetishists are male.

The object chosen as the fetish has a symbolic value, usually related to some childhood association.

Many 'normal' people use fetishistic procedures to arouse their desire, for example the female partner being asked to wear a particular type of underwear. At the other extreme are fetishists who are able to achieve satisfaction only by touching or gazing at the fetishistic object whilst masturbating.

If the fetishistic behaviour becomes a problem – either through marital conflict or court appearances – behaviour therapy may be attempted after psychotherapy (which is of limited help) has been tried.

Exhibitionism

This is an extremely common deviation. It is almost exclusively confined to males and involves the compulsive need to deliberately expose the genitals to the opposite sex in order to achieve sexual excitement. This procedure is usually accompanied or followed by masturbation. The victim's fear or surprise enhances the sexual excitement.

Physical or sexual assault is rarely a sequel, and the majority of exhibitionists are sexually inadequate individuals who are displacing their aggressive feelings towards women.

Voyeurism

This is a parallel and common deviation to exhibitionism. It involves obtaining sexual gratification by observing the sexual activity or nudity of others. It is very common in adolescents.

As with exhibitionists, the persistent voyeur ('Peeping Tom') is immature emotionally, may feel sexually inadequate and may have many unresolved conflicts.

Paedophilia

This is the sexual attraction of an adult (who may be homosexual or heterosexual) to children of the same or both sexes.

Most cases are males, and a personality disorder is almost always associated, especially traits reflecting social and sexual inadequacy and emotional deprivation in childhood.

The desires become evident in adolescence or later, and involve masturbating or merely touching the child's genitals, or inducing the child to reciprocate this behaviour to the adult. Actual intercourse is very rarely attempted.

A number of child murders result from the child's lack of cooperation, whence the paedophile's sexual frustration is manifested as aggression.

In a percentage of cases, subnormality of intelligence or brain damage are present – in these instances, there is a loss of judgement and social and sexual self-control.

Other sexual deviations are:

Frotteurism: the rubbing of an individual's genitals against a stranger – usually in crowds.

Buggery (or sodomy): the insertion of the penis into the anus of a man or woman is so common as to be regarded as normal sexual practice.

Bestiality: involves sexual intercourse with animals. It is chiefly confined to individuals living in isolated rural areas where they are deprived of the opposite sex. It is also found in psychotic or mentally retarded patients.

In general, the treatment of sexual deviations requires long term psychotherapy aimed at exploring unresolved sexual conflicts and relieving guilt feelings. The patient needs to be highly motivated for treatment. Court referrals often provide the necessary impetus for treatment.

Unfortunately, insight oriented psychotherapy is frequently of little help in altering the deviation, although anxiety may be relieved. In these instances, behaviour therapy may be tried.

In many individuals, suppression of the libido is attempted using a major tranquillizer (e.g. benperidol) or female sex hormones in males (stilboestrol 5–10 mg daily). A more recent suppressor of libido in males is the specific anti-androgen cyproterone acetate (Androcur) which at 100 mg daily in divided doses works in four or five days. The resulting drop in plasma testosterone level is reversible on stopping the drug.

Sexual behaviour is frequently, but not always, altered by the presence of certain psychological conditions.

1   Mentally retarded individuals rarely have normal heterosexual relationships. More primitive behaviour, e.g. masturbation or mutual masturbation is more common. However, minimally retarded individuals are capable of normal heterosexual relationships and even marriage. In general, their sexual behaviour tends to be somewhat disinhibited.

2 In organic syndromes, where insight and judgement are impaired, sexual behaviour is often thoughtless and uninhibited. Social control is lost to a greater or lesser degree too, and aggressiveness or hypersexuality may be found.

3 Affective disorders: a loss of libido and impotence is common in depression and anxiety states. Increased sexual desire and promiscuity is associated with hypomania.

4 In schizophrenia, a reduction in sexual drive is very common. More rarely, the reverse occurs.

5 In the neuroses: as has been discussed, unresolved childhood conflicts associated with or without personality disorder are invariably associated with psychosexual disorder.

In hysterical personalities, sexual indifference, frigidity or impotence, genital anaesthesia or inability in achieving orgasm are common, often associated with a more superficial seductive manner.

13 Psychiatry and the Law

The Mental Health Act of 1959 was a major advance in the liberalization of social and legal attitudes to the mentally ill. It was designed to introduce informality of care and simplify the mechanism of admission and legal procedures as well as the care of patients in psychiatric hospitals.

The term 'certification' was abolished and instead there are 'applications for admission' to hospital.

No documents are now required for informal admission, and hospital psychiatrists have the right to refuse the admission of a patient.

Mental hospitals have been put on the same footing as general hospitals, community care under the aegis of local authorities has been encouraged and the old definitions of mental illness have been altered and re-classified as follows:

(a) Mental disorder: meaning mental illness and any other disorder or disability of mind.

(b) Subnormality: defined as 'a state of arrested or incomplete development of mind (not amounting to severe subnormality) which includes subnormality of IQ and is of a nature or degree which requires or is susceptible to treatment'.

(c) Severe subnormality: meaning a state of arrested or incomplete development of mind including subnormality of IQ which is of such a nature or degree that the patient is incapable of living an independent life, or of guarding himself against serious exploitations, or will be so incapable when of an age to do so.

(d) Psychopathic disorder: this is defined as a persistent disorder of personality resulting in abnormally aggressive or seriously irresponsible conduct. Subnormality may or may not be present.

120

Formal admission

This can be arranged through 2 procedures:

(a) For observation.
(b) For treatment.

Application for a patient can be made by either the nearest relative or a mental welfare officer (MWO) and several forms are provided:

Form 1　　Application for admission for observation (Section 25) – 28 days duration.

Form 2　　Emergency application for admission for observation (Section 29) – 72 hours duration.

Form 4A　Application by nearest relative for admission for treatment (Section 26) – 6 months duration.

Form 4B　Application by a MWO (Section 26).

Grounds for application for observation

(a) The patient's mental disorder is such that he requires observation for a limited time.

(b) That he should be detained in the interests of his own health or safety, or with a view to the protection of others.

Grounds for application for treatment

(a) That the patient is suffering from mental disorder, either mental illness or subnormality.

(b) In cases of patients under 21, psychopathic disorder or subnormality. The disorder must be of such a degree that the detention of the patient in hospital for treatment is warranted.

(c) That the patient should be so detained in the interests of his health or safety, or for the protection of others.

Medical recommendations

1 Must be signed within 7 days of seeing the patient.
2 One of the doctors must be specially approved (under Section 28) by a local health authority as having special experience in the diagnosis and treatment of mental disorder.
3 One recommendation must be completed by a doctor who has treated and knows the patient.

4 One recommendation may be completed by a doctor on the staff of the admitting hospital, provided that it is an NHS (National Health Service) hospital.

(3 and 4 do not apply to Section 29.)

There are a number of special forms available:

Form 3A Medical recommendation for admission for observation (Section 25 or 29).

Form 3B Joint medical recommendation for admission for observation (Section 25 or 29).

Form 5A Medical recommendation for admission for treatment(Section 26).

Form 5B Joint medical recommendation for admission for treatment (Section 26).

Certain people are legally excluded from signing a medical recommendation for admission to hospital or guardianship:

(a) The applicant.
(b) A partner of the applicant or of a doctor who may be making the other recommendation.
(c) A person employed as an assistant by the applicant or by the doctor making the other recommendation.
(d) A person who receives or who has interest in the receipt of any payments made on account of the maintenance of the patient.
(e) If one medical recommendation is signed by a hospital doctor, no other member of the staff may sign the second recommendation.

Emergency admissions

In an emergency, either a doctor or a nurse can make an application for urgent admission (on a Section 29). A second medical recommendation must then be obtained within 72 hours of admission to a hospital, or the compulsory detention lapses.

A Section 30 applies to patients already in hospital, and is usually completed by the responsible medical officer. It is otherwise like a Section 29.

A Section 135 enables a police officer to enter any premises if it is suspected that a person suffering from mental disorder is being ill treated, neglected or unable to care for himself.

A Section 136 enables a police officer to remove an individual to a hospital for observation for a period of 72 hours.

Discharge after absence without leave

Patients who are compulsorily detained and who absent themselves without leave must be discharged after 28 days if they are on a treatment order and after 6 months absence if they are detained because they are subnormal or psychopathic.

There are also specific recommendations in the new Act for the humane treatment of patients by nurses and the procedures for dealing with accidents and injuries.

Guardianship

This is given on the grounds that an individual:

(a) suffers with mental illness or subnormality
(b) or psychopathic disorder or subnormality if under 21 and that the nature or degree of the disorder warrants reception into guardianship and is necessary for the protection of the patient and/or others.

Two medical recommendations must accompany the application. The rules are similar as those for treatment and observation orders. Guardianship is for a period of one year, renewable for a year and then for two year periods until the age of 25.

Appeals

Mental Health Review Tribunals were set up with lay, professional and medical members. They have the power to discharge patients from hospital and rescind the order that he was admitted on, if they are satisfied he is not dangerous and does not suffer from the condition he was admitted for.

The **law in Scotland** is essentially the same; the main differences are:

1 An independent Mental Welfare Board was set up, exercising protective functions over the mentally disabled.
2 It has powers to supervise all aspects of mental illness,

treatment, detention and discharge, and to initiate the investing of appeals for wrongful detention, as there is no Mental Health Review Tribunal.

3 Compulsory applications are dealt with as in England, except that a lay person in the form of a Sheriff must approve all applications for them to become effective.

4 All forms of subnormality are described as mental disorder.

5 The durations of compulsory detention differ.

Court of protection

Its function is to manage the property and affairs of people unable to do so themselves because of mental disorder. A receiver is appointed by a court who acts on the patient's behalf. This is initiated by the court after receiving a medical opinion on the patient under **Section 101** of the Mental Health Act, 1959. The majority of patients involved are disorientated or demented.

Testamentary capacity

This is the ability of an individual to make a will. He must:

1 Know he is making a will and what this implies.

2 Know the nature and extent of his property.

3 Know the people who have claims on his bounty.

4 Have sufficient judgement and insight that he can determine the relative strengths of the claims of his relatives and friends.

5 The presence of gross mental disorder is not incompatible with making a will unless, for example, paranoid delusions are present, directed against a reasonable claimant.

The Homicide Act, the McNaghton rules and diminished responsibility

The legal concept of 'soundness of mind' takes for granted the principle that an individual is accountable for his actions.

Prior to the Homicide Act of 1957, mental disorder in relation to crime was assessed by the **McNaghton rules.** They were established in 1843 following the trial of the individual who murdered Sir Robert Peel's secretary. He was found to be paranoid, deluded and insane, and was sentenced to incarceration in a mental asylum.

The criteria of the McNaghton rules were very strict and in many ways unfair. The rules stated that an individual could only be excused his crime if:

1 He did not know what he was doing when he committed the crime.
2 He did know it, but did not know that he was doing wrong.

In practice, the rules only applied to grossly psychotic or subnormal individuals.

The new Homicide Act of 1957

This Act recognized the concept of **diminished responsibility,** so that, for example, a person accused of murder could have the charge reduced to manslaughter because of the presence of mental disorder.

Courts are now more prepared to take into account motivation, personality disorders and mood changes.

In many instances, if 'diminished responsibility' is accepted by the court, the individual may not be tried at all, or if found guilty is recommended to have psychiatric treatment as an outpatient, or in a psychiatric hospital voluntarily or compulsorily.

Despite this liberalization of the laws, there are still many controversial issues, for example, patients who have hysterical amnesia or a post epileptic automatism, who, after committing a crime, later deny all knowledge of it.

Part 5 of the Act allows for the remand in custody of the accused in order to obtain a medical or psychiatric report.

Detention of criminals in mental hospitals

Section 60 allows a court to transfer a convicted criminal to a psychiatric hospital if:

(a) It is satisfied on the written or oral evidence of two doctors that the patient suffers from mental disorder, psychopathic disorder or severe subnormality of a nature or degree warranting detention for the purpose of treatment or reception into guardianship.
(b) It is satisfied that a Section 60 is the most suitable method of disposal, after considering the nature of the offence and the patient's personality.
(c) The patient must be hospitalized within 28 days. The patient is

detainable in a hospital for one year, but is dischargeable earlier by the doctor under whose care he falls.

Section 65 is similar to Section 60 but there are special restrictions concerning discharge without a time limit. Many patients on this section are detained in high security hospitals, e.g. Broadmoor.

Section 72 allows for the transfer of a prisoner from prison to a psychiatric hospital for treatment with similar provisions as on a Section 60/65.

Malingering

Psychiatrists are frequently asked in court, especially in cases of compensation, to distinguish between malingering and hysteria in a claimed disability, physical or mental.

By malingering is meant the imitation of disease or disability which is not present, or the gross exaggeration of a minor disability and its deliberate attribution to an accident that did not, in fact, cause it, for personal advantage.

It is extremely difficult to differentiate between malingering and hysteria.

Imitation of illness may be indicated by:

(a) The possibility of financial gain.
(b) A trivial injury resulting in severe or prolonged disablement.
(c) The disability being one that can be imitated.
(d) A situation when the complaint does not conform to a recognized organic pattern.

Psychiatry and crime

There is no easily defined or reliable picture of the typical criminal.

Criminal acts are determined by the legal code. What is a crime in one country or culture might be acceptable as normal social behaviour in another.

Most studies of criminals demonstrate the importance of psychological motivation. It is invariably a complex interreaction between personality, emotional state, intelligence, education, socioeconomic and cultural background.

The majority of offenders are male. 50% of all offences in the UK are committed by youths under 21 and they have several features in common. They tend to be of low IQ or educational subnormality, underachieve educationally and come from emotionally and economically deprived homes. Crime is more prevalent in the lower social classes in families where social mobility, overcrowding and lack of parental guidance is present.

50% of persistently aggressive or violent offenders have abnormal EEGs (electroencephalograms).

Only a small percentage of criminals (10%–15%) require specific psychiatric treatment. The psychiatrist does, however, play an important part in the assessment and rehabilitation of offenders within prison and many prisons are now treatment orientated.

2%–3% of offenders are mentally ill. They range from psychotics (manic depressive and schizophrenic) to subnormality and epilepsy.

A further percentage are classified as **sociopathic.** This implies that they have personality disorders, are persistently antisocial, and behave in a callous, aggressive, egocentric way. Their behaviour is impulsive and immature, and out of context to the provocation. They do not learn by experience and respond poorly to advice or treatment of any kind.

Another important group of criminals are drug takers and alcoholics. The former tend to be adolescents or in their twenties. Their crimes involve the forging of prescriptions, and the theft of drugs or money in order to purchase drugs.

In the middle aged and elderly, the first evidence of personality change due to organic brain disease, e.g. arteriosclerotic dementia or syphilis, may be antisocial behaviour.

14 Making a Diagnosis in Psychiatry

The way in which a diagnosis is made can be illustrated by imagining a female patient presenting to a doctor and complaining of palpitations. She also suffers from shakiness, muscular tension, apprehension and excessive perspiration. It will come to mind that she may be suffering from an **anxiety state.** It would be dangerous to jump to this conclusion at this stage without asking further questions. Suppose that as the interview continues she also confesses that she is in low spirits, has lost her energy, feels hopeless, has lost a lot of weight through lack of appetite, wakes early in the morning and suffers from suicidal ideas. Now the doctor will argue that the most likely diagnosis seems to be that of a depressive illness (in which anxiety symptoms are known to be quite common).

He will change his ideas quite radically if she goes on to say that she hears hallucinatory voices addressing her in the third person and feels that all her actions are controlled by a mysterious machine located in the basement. In fact he may be convinced that she suffers from schizophrenia. This diagnosis would be acceptable as long as it were established that she suffered from a functional mental illness. However, **any** psychological symptom can be produced by organic brain disease. It would therefore be necessary to exclude the presence of brain disease before her particular hallucinations and passivity delusions were accepted as proof of schizophrenia.

We now know that any neurotic symptom can be produced by a psychosis. A diagnosis of neurotic illness is therefore made partly by the demonstration of positive evidence **for** the diagnosis, and partly by exclusion of any more serious and fundamental disorder. We can now draw up a list of classes of diagnosis in rank order (descending degree of severity) as follows:

Neurosis.
Affective psychosis.
Schizophrenia.
Organic brain syndrome.

At any level we consider the disorders below as being important in the **differential diagnosis.** That is to say they have to be considered as serious contenders for the final diagnosis.

To show this more clearly, let us suppose that we suspect a particular patient of suffering from an affective psychosis (e.g. depressive psychosis). If we come across features of **neurosis** this will not alter our opinion. If, however, we come across features of schizophrenia or organic brain syndrome we shall have to think again. This is an important aspect of psychiatric diagnosis that has only recently been given adequate recognition.

It is possible to make the rank order of diagnoses even more elaborate if so desired. For instance most **other** neurotic features can be found in depressive neurosis, so it might be possible to list depressive neurosis below the other neurotic illnesses. Similarly most of the features of the acute organic brain syndrome and of the dysmnestic syndrome may be found in the chronic organic brain syndrome, so maybe this last condition should be put bottom of all.

These refinements are somewhat debatable and unnecessary for most purposes. It is enough if the general principle is accepted that positive evidence is not sufficient for most psychiatric diagnoses to be made.

Another diagnostic pitfall is the relationship between personality and illness. This has been touched on when discussing the diagnosis of hysteria (see pp. 16–20). A patient with, say, an anxiety state may be falsely diagnosed as having a hysterical illness if she is attention-seeking, manipulative, histrionic, egocentric and vain. Here the **personality** qualities of the patient have overwhelmed the doctor and have made him think vaguely of 'hysteria' without being precise enough in distinguishing the illness from the personality.

In fact there is an association between illnesses and personalities of the same name. That is to say, obsessional personalities are prone to obsessional illnesses, hysterical personalities tend to get hysterical symptoms and so on. But the associations are not so strong as to be exclusive. Obsessional personalities often get depressive illnesses and may even get hysteria. Hysterical personalities may develop schizophrenia. **Any personality type may develop any mental illness.**

15 The Aetiology of Mental Disorder

Aetiology is the study of the causes of disease. In this section we will look at such possible causes as infection, physical injury, heredity, poisoning, childhood upbringing, unpleasant events in adult life and abnormal diet.

Visible disease of the brain can cause any symptom that is found in mental illness (see pp. 7–11). The cause is obvious when a *physical injury* produces the brain damage. With a severe injury in adult life many intellectual faculties are lost and the patient may end up as **demented** (see pp. 66–68). With an injury producing less damage the intellectual impairment may not be so obvious as the change in behaviour, producing the features of **personality disorder.** If brain injury occurs during the birth of the patient it will show itself later either as personality disorder or as **mental handicap** (see pp. 89–98). With damage limited to one small part of the brain **epilepsy** can result (see pp. 74–76).

Infections cause the acute organic brain syndrome or **delirium** (see pp. 63–65). If they cause permanent destruction of brain tissue the chronic organic brain syndrome or **dementia** results (see pp. 66–68). The most famous example in psychiatry has been the disease caused by syphilis known as general paralysis of the insane (GPI), because this was the first mental illness for which a specific cause was discovered. It is rare nowadays.

Amphetamine psychosis is a clear example of a mental illness caused by *poisoning*. The illness is indistinguishable in its symptoms from **paranoid schizophrenia** (see pp. 53–54) and occurs when amphetamine addicts take large quantities of this or a related drug. Other drugs can cause **delirium,** especially those with atropine-like actions. Hallucinogenic drugs such as LSD cause a picture with features of either delirium or of functional psychosis. **Alcohol** is probably the commonest poison in the sense used here. Apart from the obvious intoxication and the problem of alcoholism as a disorder in itself (see pp. 78–80), excessive use of alcohol contributes to the cause of various psychiatric disorders. In some cases it goes as far as producing **dementia**. A more restricted degree of damage produces Korsakoff's psychosis (see pp. 65–66) in which recent memory is particularly affected. **Withdrawal** of alcohol from someone regularly taking large quantities can produce **delirium tremens** (see pp. 64–65). **Delirium tremens** is one possible withdrawal syndrome to a number of other addicting drugs, including barbiturates, chloral and methaqualone (see pp. 64–65).

Psychiatric disorder is produced by *deficiency of some vitamins* (e.g. in pellagra) but the diet in most of the developed countries is usually not so inadequate as to do this in the ordinary way. In general, serious deficiencies do not develop unless the behaviour of the patient is in some way unusual, so that vitamin deficiency is as likely to be the **result** of mental disorder as the cause of it. Alcoholism is a good example. The alcoholic may neglect his diet, and in any case the metabolism burns up available vitamin B_1 (thiamin, aneurin) in the body. Deficiency of this vitamin leads to the **Korsakoff's psychosis** mentioned above. A similar picture can result from deficiency of vitamin B_{12} (cyanocobalamin), which can arise in turn from disorders of the gastrointestinal tract or after gastrectomy. Drug therapy (e.g. for epilepsy) may give rise to deficiency of folic acid.

Disorders of the endocrine system can produce psychiatric disturbance. Hyperthyroidism produces a picture mimicking an **anxiety state** and hypothyroidism produces impaired intellectual function. Otherwise rises and falls in the blood levels of hormones (including not only thyroid hormone but also those produced by the adrenal and other glands) may trigger off psychological reactions which range from **depressive illness** (of merely neurotic degree) through **affective psychoses** to **schizophrenic-like illnesses,** often paranoid in type.

The commonest forms of *organic brain disease* are **senile dementia** and **arteriosclerotic dementia** (see pp. 66–68). The cause is usually described as 'degenerative' but this does not tell us much except that they arise in old age. Diabetes, hypertension and high blood fat levels all make one more likely to develop arteriosclerosis. The pathology of senile dementia is similar to that of **Alzheimer's disease** (see pp. 67–68), one of the presenile dementias in which heredity seems to play some part.

Among organic brain disease the role of *heredity* is most easily seen in **Huntington's chorea** (see p. 68). This is carried as a dominant gene, so that half of the offspring of an affected parent will be expected to develop the disease. Among mental illnesses this is exceptional, despite the common view that insanity is hereditary. Of course there is **some** truth in this idea. A child born to a patient with schizophrenia or manic–depressive psychosis has a one in ten chance (or possibly more) of developing the same illness himself. This does not mean that we shall never find ways of cutting down the incidence of these disorders. Even with Huntington's chorea the fact that the age of onset varies considerably from case to case suggests that if we could control the factors that **delayed** the onset then we would be well on the way to preventing the disease altogether.

In the vast majority of patients attending the psychiatric clinic we do not expect to find evidence of infection, poisoning, brain disease, or brain trauma and there is usually no strong hereditary history. So what are the causes of psychiatric disorder that remain? It seems reasonable to accept that *early childhood experience* plays an important part in influencing the way the mind works. This is especially so in the formation of the person's **personality** or character make-up (see pp. 84–88). It may also be expected to be at least partly responsible for the weaknesses that he shows to certain forms of stress. In psychoanalytical terms the personality disorder is said to represent **fixation** at a certain period of development. When the patient succumbs to psychological stress later on, the illness he develops shows a **regression** back to the corresponding infantile period of development. For example the person who is **fixated** at the oral level of development may show a number of character traits of dependence (see pp. 85–86) whether relying on other people or on drugs. If under severe stress he **regresses** back to the oral phase he may show complete helplessness, requiring nurses to perform even the simplest task for him, as if he were a baby again.

This psychoanalytical model illustrates the general idea that a person is **predisposed** to develop a psychiatric illness (whether from heredity or from early upbringing) and that at a later time events occur (*'psychological trauma'*) that **precipitate** the illness.

What sort of events can do this? Single events such as bereavement, loss of job, loss of status, loss of role (e.g. when a woman loses her role as mother as her children leave home) and disappointments can all trigger off distress that in turn causes mental disorder if the affected person is unable to deal with his feelings in an adaptive way. Often a patient gives a history of **several** calamities in the year or so before his breakdown. When unpleasant things have happened to us we get **depressed.** When there is the threat of unpleasant things that **may** happen to us the reaction is one of **anxiety.** If something very frightening happens **(or there is an intolerable situation causing much emotional stress)** the patient may resolve the situation by developing **hysteria** (see pp. 16–20), or he may displace his anxiety into the superficially meaningless rituals of **obsessions** (see pp. 14–16).

The precipitating factor may not be a discrete, separate shock but rather the unpleasant situation in which the patient finds himself daily. It has been shown that one of the reasons for **relapse** in schizophrenia is the patient entering a highly charged emotional atmosphere (maybe his parental home) where he is continually subjected to critical comments. It seems possible that such a situation could also produce the breakdown in the first place.

Attempts to get evidence for the environmental factors that are concerned in the production of schizophrenia have sometimes been disappointing. **Epidemiology** is the study of the distribution of disease in the community. Two of the main discoveries made about schizophrenia have been that it is associated with poverty or unskilled work (social class V) and that it occurs especially in the centre of cities. These findings on the distribution of schizophrenia looked at first as if they meant that slum conditions produced the disease. It has now been shown that this is probably not the explanation.

The social class trend affects **prevalence** (the **total** number of cases) rather than **incidence** (the number of **new** cases in a given time). Also the parents of the patients have a social class distribution that does not show the excess in social class V. It looks as if the patients were born into average homes, but then drifted down the social scale as they became schizophrenic. It is in social class V where these patients are found eventually rather than where they occur initially.

Within the centre of cities, the latest research suggests that the hospital admissions for schizophrenia are excessive not especially for the long term residents of the district, but among those that have recently arrived. It appears that the cause of the increased admission rate is the tendency of schizophrenic patients to drift into the city centre (e.g. to common lodging houses) prior to their breakdown.

It can be seen that both of these epidemiological findings tell us not so much about the cause of schizophrenia as about its effects.

It is widely accepted that psychological trauma can precipitate neurotic illnesses. The part that environmental stress plays in the production of the functional psychoses (schizophrenia and manic-depressive psychosis) is more likely to be disputed. The reason for this disagreement is that although the functional psychoses are not associated with visible organic disease it is likely that **chemical** changes in the brain are involved in their chain of causation. There are various pieces of evidence for this. We have seen how high doses of amphetamine can produce the picture of schizophrenia. A classical depressive psychosis can result from treatment with the drug reserpine. Both of these drugs are thought to act by altering the effect of neurotransmitter substances – chemicals that pass the messages on from one nerve cell to the next. Drugs that relieve depression interfere with the action of two of the neurotransmitters in particular – noradrenaline and serotonin (5-hydroxytryptamine or 5HT). Drugs that improve schizophrenia do the same for another neurotransmitter (dopamine).

If we accept that functional psychoses are accompanied by chemical changes in the brain, the important question that remains is: What causes the chemical changes in the first place? One possible way to look at the evidence is to take the view that environmental stress and worrying events cause the brain to **alter its pattern of function,** and that this altered function in turn leads to changes in the turnover of neurotransmitter substances. For the time being we can say that in the search for the causes of mental illness discoveries are being made every year that goes by, but it will be some time before we can work out exactly what they all imply for purposes of treatment and prevention.

16 Epidemiology of Mental Illness

Sudden outbreaks of illness (epidemics) are becoming rarer in western society and epidemiologists are devoting themselves rather to the study of how illnesses are distributed in the community, and why there are higher rates for illness in some occupations and in certain localities.

The term 'prevalence' refers to the **total number** of cases of a disorder in a given population. The term 'incidence' refers to the number of **new cases** that arise in a specified period of time (e.g. one year).

Social class

It is customary to describe social class in the following terms:

Social class I	The professions
Social class II	Supervisors and managers
Social class III	Skilled workers
Social class IV	Semi-skilled workers
Social class V	Unskilled workers

Using this scheme an excess of patients with psychoses has been found in the lower social classes. Schizophrenia is found particularly in social class V. This finding is most marked for **prevalence**.

Geographical distribution

Faris and Dunham (1939) in Chicago showed that the incidence of mental illness as determined by hospital admission was higher in the centre of the city. They found paranoid schizophrenia in the rooming house immigrant areas. Alcoholism, senile and arteriosclerotic psychoses were associated to the percentage of the population on relief (social security benefits). High rates for

135

schizophrenia from the city centre have been found in this country by Hare (1956) among male first admissions at Bristol.

Other factors

In addition, epidemiological studies have suggested increased rates of psychiatric illness with **isolation, residential mobility, occupational class mobility**, especially downward, and the **separated, divorced, widowed and single**, though not all of these findings have been confirmed in further studies.

Rates for alcoholism have been found to be high for **low socioeconomic status, residential mobility, class and occupational mobility, widowers, divorced and separated**, and certain **religions** and races, e.g. Irish Roman Catholics; the rates for Jews are low.

Rates for senile and arteriosclerotic dementia have been shown to be high in central areas in the USA, but not in the UK.

Interpretation of the findings on schizophrenia

The above findings could be explained in at least two ways. Firstly that schizophrenia, or the tendency to it, could cause the decline in social class position and the migration to poor housing conditions. On the other hand, it might be that being born into a poor family and living in slum conditions might increase the risk of developing schizophrenia. Two studies have helped to clarify this position. Dunham (1965) investigated two subcommunities within Detroit that had different social characteristics and different rates for mental illness. One district had an incidence of schizophrenia three times that of the other. When cases resident in the community for 5 years and over are counted, the rates for schizophrenia prove to be identical. The conclusion appears to be that since recent arrivals account for the excess, it is the drift to these areas of affected individuals that is important rather than any effect of living in the particular area. Goldberg and Morrison (1963) looking at schizophrenics admitted to hospital 'found that the patients showed the expected concentration in unskilled jobs, but their fathers appeared to represent a typical occupational sample of the population'. 'The father's occupation at the time of the patient's birth (obtained from the recorded details of each patient at birth) was determined for male patients on first admissions to mental hospitals with a diagnosis of schizophrenia and compared with that of the patient at the time of admission. The sample was drawn from admissions in 1956 of men aged 20–34 years (to correspond with the age group of their fathers when the patients were born).'

Since the fathers had a social class pattern just like that of the ordinary population, one cannot say that the patients had grown up in particularly poor surroundings. Rather they had slipped down the social scale because – probably as a **result** of their illness – they were able to cope only with relatively unskilled work.

In both these examples (centres of cities, social class) the high rates that are found seem to be the result of **drift** of patients into that part of society. The environmental effect in the **cause** of schizophrenia probably lies in more subtle relationships (see pp. 46–47).

17 *Physical Methods of Treatment*

In the last twenty-five years, there have been significant and revolutionary advances in the treatment of mental illness.

Electroconvulsive therapy (ECT) was introduced for the treatment of depression; surgical operations on the brain (leucotomy and stereotactic procedures) have been devised to relieve aggression, tension and depression, and psychotherapy and social therapy in hospitals and in the community have been intensively expanded and re-evaluated.

The simultaneous introduction of rapidly effective and reasonably safe tranquillizers, antidepressant and anti-psychotic drugs, has introduced a dynamism into treatment that had been, for decades before, static, custodial, and pessimistically non-productive.

A vast array of new psychotropic drugs becomes available every year, and it is difficult for the beginner in psychiatry to make an easy evaluation of them, or indeed to need know their pharmacological properties in detail.

In principle, it is wisest to learn the clinical usage of two or three drugs in each of the main groups; tranquillizers, antidepressants, and antipsychotics, and to reserve the use of the others to a specialist.

Classification of psychotropic drugs

1	Neuroleptics (major tranquillizers)	Phenothiazines Butyrophenones Thioxanthenes Reserpine
2	Anxiolytics (minor tranquillizers)	Benzodiazepines

3	Hypnotics/sedatives	Barbiturates
		Alcohol
		Chloral hydrate
		Methaqualone

4	Antidepressants	Tricyclic
		Tetracyclic
		Monoamine oxidase inhibitors
		(MAOIs)

5	Miscellaneous	Disulfiram
		Citrated calcium carbimide
		Vitamins
		Lithium salts
		Propranolol
		Amphetamines

The major tranquillizers

Most phenothiazine and non-phenothiazine neuroleptics have **similar pharmacological actions**.

They have a central adrenergic blocking action and diminish the emotional response to external and internal stimuli by their effects on the three major integrating systems of the brain. That is, they stimulate the amygdaloid nuclei and the limbic system, and they depress the hypothalmus and reticular activating system.

They all produce:

1 A special type of sedation – apathy and drowsiness with relatively little clouding of consciousness.
2 Parasympathetic blockade (atropinic) effects – a dry mouth, dilated pupils, blurred vision and constipation.
3 Adrenergic blockade effects – vasodilatation, a drop in blood pressure and postural hypotension, with a decreased body temperature.
4 Endocrinal effects – increased production of prolactin sometimes results in the stimulation of lactation, even if the individual is not pregnant.
5 Extrapyramidal effects – e.g. tremor and stiffness of the limbs, **akathisia** (motor restlessness) and **dyskinesia** (muscle spasm). **Anti-parkinsonian** drugs are sometimes given concomitantly

when major tranquillizers are prescribed.
6　They are convulsants in very large doses.
7　Photosensitivity of the skin commonly occurs.
8　Skin pigmentation occurs after long usage.
9　Allergic subjects sometimes develop cholestatic jaundice.
10　Eye changes (retinal pigmentation and opacities in the lens and cornea) occur if high doses are used for long periods of time (with thioridazine mainly).

Major tranquillizers are used:

(a)　To control excitement, agitation and aggression in psychotic patients, demented patients and subnormal individuals.
(b)　To suppress delusions and hallucinations.
(c)　Less frequently, as anti-pruritics and anti-emetics.
(d)　In the treatment of drug and alcohol withdrawal symptoms.
(e)　They are sometimes used in small doses, to control anxiety and agitation in the psychoneuroses.

The average daily doses are shown in Table 1.
In acutely excited patients, daily doses of up to 1000–1500 mg – for example: chlorpromazine (orally) or 4–600 mg i.m. may be given, or haloperidol 40–80 mg (orally) or 10–40 mg i.m. or i.v.

Phenothiazines

It is wisest to get to know two or three phenothiazines well rather than experiment with the vast number that are available. Chlorpromazine and thioridazine are probably among the most widely used. After initial stabilization, patients (especially schizophrenics) may be kept on maintenance dosage for many years.

The piperazine group have more stimulant effects and are given in smaller doses. They also have more powerful extrapyramidal side effects. Trifluoperazine is the best known member of this group. It is especially useful in apathetic inert schizophrenics.

The long acting major tranquillizers (fluphenazine enanthate and decanoate; flupenthixol decanoate) are a major advance, especially in the outpatient management of unreliable patients who neither take the oral medication prescribed or attend as outpatients regularly. The dose has a prolonged therapeutic effect for 2–4 weeks and is usually given in special clinics by a community nurse.

Pimozide has stimulant properties and need only be given in one

TABLE 1 The major tranquillizers

Phenothiazines		Trade name	Daily dose (oral) (mg)
Aliphatic	chlorpromazine	Largactil	75–1000
	promazine	Sparine	75–1000
	fluopromazine	Vespral	25–150
	methotrimeprazine	Veractil	25–500
Piperidine	thioridazine	Melleril	50–1000
	pericyazine	Neulactil	10–90
Piperazine	trifluoperazine	Stelazine	5–50
	prochlorperazine	Stemetil	15–100
	perphenazine	Fentazine	6–60
	fluphenazine-enanthate	Moditen-enanthate	12.5–25 i.m. every 2–4 weeks
	fluphenazine-decanoate	Modecate	12.5–25 i.m. every 2–4 weeks
	fluphenazine	Moditen	2.5–1.0
	thiopropozate	Dartalan	15–100

Non-phenothiazines

Butyrophenones			
	haloperidol	Serenace	2–40
	trifluoperidol	Triperidol	0.5–2
Thioxanthenes			
	chlorprothixene	Taracten	30–90
	thiotrixene	Navane	10–30
	flupenthixol-decanoate	Depixol	20–40 i.m.
	reserpine	Serpasil	0.25–5.0
	tetrabenzine	Nitoman	30–150
	diphenyl-butylpiperidine	Pimozide (ORAP)	2–8

N.B. A student would not be expected to memorize this table in detail

daily dose. It has few extrapyramidal or autonomic side effects.

Rauwolfia alkaloids (e.g. Serpasil) are rarely used because of their hypotensive effects and because they rapidly produce severe depression.

Butyrophenones may be used interchangeably with the phenothiazines or combined with them. They are thought to exert their action via blockage of dopamine receptors in the brain and have more potent extrapyramidal side effects than the phenothiazines.

Other non-phenothiazine tranquillizers are occasionally used.

Minor tranquillizers (anxiolytics)

The term 'minor tranquillizer' has been replaced by 'anxiolytic' (anxiety reducer), as the drugs in this group are neither minor, nor have much in common with the major tranquillizers.

Barbiturates are now rarely used as tranquillizers and have been superseded by the benzodiazepines.

The benzodiazepines are extremely safe tranquillizers: their toxicity is low, only very large doses are lethal, and addiction or physical dependence is uncommon.

Side effects are also minimal. The most common are drowsiness, ataxia, headache, impaired judgement, and confusion in the elderly or demented. Although they potentiate most psychotropic drugs, especially alcohol, they may be given safely with any antidepressant drug.

There is little to choose between the many benzodiazepines available. Benzodiazepines are chiefly used to reduce anxiety in the psychoneuroses and in other illnesses where anxiety or agitation is present (Table 2).

TABLE 2

Benzodiazepine	Trade name	Daily dose range (mg)
chlordiazepoxide	Librium	5–60
diazepam	Valium	5–30
oxazepam	Serenid D	15–60
medazapam	Nobrium	10–40
lorazepam	Ativan	1–5
potassium chlorazepate	Tranxene	15–45
nitrazepam	Mogadon	5–15
flurazepam	Dalmane	15–45
temazepam	Euhypnos	10–20

They are also used to control withdrawal symptoms in drug addiction and alcoholism, and as anticonvulsants in the treatment of epilepsy. They may be given intravenously or intramuscularly (especially diazepam) to control rapidly all types of excitement, agitation, and status epilepticus.

Nitrazepam is a widely used safe hypnotic night sedative, and flurazepam is an alternative.

Meprobamate (Equanil, 400–1200 mg daily) has also been replaced by the benzodiazepines. It is about as effective as the barbiturates. Dependence rapidly develops and it has many side effects (skin rashes, headache, ataxia, gastrointestinal upset). Meprobamate is dangerous in overdosage and as little as 16 g can be fatal.

Benzoctamine (Tacitin) has properties similar to the benzodiazepines, but is rarely used.

Major tranquillizers when given in small doses, act as anxiolytics. They might be given to patients for whom routine anxiolytics had proved to be ineffective.

Some tricyclic antidepressants, especially amitryptiline and dothiepin, have anxiolytic properties and are used when anxiety and depression co-exist.

Alcohol remains the most common anxiolytic used by the general public.

Hypnotics and sedatives

Barbiturates, although effective hypnotics or sedatives which depress the central nervous system, have been displaced in the treatment of anxiety and insomnia by the benzodiazepines for a number of reasons.

Although sensitivity to barbiturates is rare, the latitude between a therapeutic dose and the production of mild toxic symptoms is very small. They result in confusion in the elderly, may aggravate depression, and rapidly produce dependence.

A significant percentage of deaths due to accidental or deliberate overdoses are found to be caused by barbiturates.

The sudden cessation of their use in large doses produces **withdrawal** symptoms such as anxiety, nausea, tremor, convulsions and delirium (see Chapter 8).

A dose over 800 mg daily easily produces confusion, vertigo and ataxia. There have been several epidemics (in the UK) of intravenous barbiturate abuse in recent years.

Dependence develops rapidly if the daily dose exceeds 1500 mg.

Short acting barbiturates given intravenously (sodium pentothal and sodium methohexitone) are used as abreactive agents, to assist in relaxation during deconditioning regimes, and as short acting anaesthetics.

All barbiturates are contraindicated in porphyria, myxoedema and liver disease.

There are three groups of barbiturates:

1   Long acting (phenobarbitone): chiefly used in the treatment of epilepsy in doses of 60–180 mg daily.

2   Medium acting amylobarbitone (amytal): 60–180 mg daily, used as an anxiolytic; amylbarbitone sodium (sodium amytal), 2–400 mg at night, used as a hypnotic; pentobarbitone (nembutal), 1–200 mg at night, used as a hypnotic.

3   Short acting quinalbarbitone (seconal): 1–200 mg at night used as a hypnotic.

In general, small doses of barbiturates are **sedative**, and large doses **hypnotic**.

Bromides are no longer used because of their side effects (skin eruptions and confusional states).

Paraldehyde is a relatively safe, quick acting hypnotic, especially if given intramuscularly (i.m.). It is infrequently used because of its unpleasant odour, and because the large volumes required by injection are painful and may cause abscess formation. The dose is 10–15 ml (oral) or 10 ml i.m.

Chloral hydrate is a relatively safe and effective alternative hypnotic. Chemically related drugs, for example tricloryl, can be given in a tablet form. Long usage produces constipation and physical dependence.

Mandrax (methaqualone 250 mg in combination with diphenhydramine hydrochloride 25 mg) is no longer used as a hypnotic because it is addictive, and produces confusional states, limb and facial paraesthesiae, and sometimes severe headaches.

Chlormethiazole (Heminevrin) is used as a sedative in the withdrawal phase of drug addiction and alcoholism (5–10 g daily, orally or i.v.). Dependence on it is recorded, but is unusual, and there are few side effects (sneezing, headache, diarrhoea).

The treatment of insomnia

Where possible the cause of the insomnia should be treated. This may be an intense emotion incompatible with sleep (e.g. burning resentment). A common cause is depressive illness, but it has been claimed that tricyclic antidepressants relieve insomnia even when the remainder of the depressive syndrome is absent.

When symptomatic drug treatment is required the most commonly used are the benzodiazepines, e.g. nitrazepam (Mogadon) 5–15 mg at night, or flurazepam (Dalmane) 15–45 mg at night. These have the advantage over the older hypnotics (mentioned above) or alcohol that physical dependence is much less likely to occur and that they are relatively safe even when taken in an overdose.

Even more attractive from the point of view of dependence is the phenothiazine group. For instance thioridazine (Melleril, Mellaril) in doses of 25–100 mg at night often produces a satisfactory night's sleep, and is free not only from physical dependence but is also unlikely to cause troublesome psychological dependence. At this daily dose toxic effects are extremely unlikely.

Antidepressants

Amphetamine derivatives (Benzedrine, Dexedrine) increase alertness, and produce euphoria, increased energy and a reduction in appetite. They were used extensively for the treatment of depression prior to the introduction of MAOIs and tricyclic antidepressants. They are rarely used today because:

1 They rapidly produce dependence (physiological and psychological) and tolerance always occurs so that increasing doses are required to produce the same effect.
2 Their effect in the treatment of severe depression is marginal.
3 Long usage in large doses produces an **amphetamine psychosis**.

Their use sometimes continues to be justified in middle aged people who have been taking small doses for many years and who find themselves unable to cope without.

They are also used in the treatment of narcolepsy, hyperkinetic behaviour in children and as an abreactive agent intravenously.

Some related stimulants are still used to treat obesity by reducing the appetite, e.g. fenfluramine (Ponderax), phenmetrazine (Preludin), methylphenidate (Ritalin). Most have similar properties, actions and disadvantages to the amphetamines.

Tricyclic antidepressants

This group of drugs are a major advance in the treatment of depression. Although more effective in the management of 'endogenous' type depressions, they are also effective in all other types of depression. Their use has reduced the frequency with which ECT is used and the number of ECT required if given simultaneously. They are rarely combined with MAOIs.

The individual dosage varies a great deal; larger doses are required when barbiturates are given simultaneously (they increase the breakdown rate of tricyclics) and smaller doses when phenothiazines are given (they decrease the breakdown rate of tricyclics).

Tricyclic antidepressants take 10–14 days to exert their action, and have maximal effects within 4–6 weeks. They should be continued for a minimum of 2–4 months after full remission as depression may redevelop if they are stopped.

They are best given 50% by day and 50% at night.

Some patients on large doses need hospitalization because of the frequency of **side effects**.

Some side effects are due to cholinergic blockade (e.g. a dry mouth, blurred vision, constipation and aggravation of glaucoma). In addition, drowsiness, agitation, tachycardia, hypotension, sweating, and a fine tremor of the limbs may occur.

Confusion and epileptiform convulsions are rarer complications.

Heart block and cardiac arrhythmias may occur in overdosage or in the presence of existing heart disease.

Acute toxicity is usually due to an overdose. It produces coma, convulsions and hyperpyrexia, in addition to the cardiac effects.

Tricyclic (iminodibenzyl) antidepressants

The iminodibenzyl series as a whole has significant **anticholinergic** effects. Trimipramine and amitriptyline have significant **sedative effects**.

Better effects are sometimes achieved by combining two antidepressants, from sub-groups A, B or C.

Dothiepin appears to be the most effective drug in group C.

Tricyclic antidepressants probably increase the stimulation of one nerve cell by another in the brain by increasing the amount of

TABLE 3

		Trade name	Average daily dose (mg)
A	imipramine	Tofranil	25–200
	desipramine	Pertofran	25–200
	trimipramine	Surmontil	25–200
	clomipramine	Anafranil	25–200
B	amitryptyline	Tryptizol	25–200
		Saroten	
		Laroxyl	
		Domical	
	protyptiline	Concordin	15–60
	nortryptiline	Aventyl	25–200
		Allegron	
C	iprindole	Prondol	45–135
	dothiepin	Prothiaden	50–200
	doxepin	Sinequan	30–300
	dibenzepin	Noveril	80–400

transmitter substance (e.g. amines) available at the nerve junction. The exact mechanism of relieving depression is not known.

Novel antidepressants

Several new antidepressants have been introduced in which the molecule is different from the typical tricyclic structure. Their place in treatment is yet to be fully assessed. Maprotiline (Ludiomil) has effects fairly similar to those of the tricyclics but possible advantages include early onset of action or relative safety (25–150 mg daily). The four ring structure of mianserin (Bolvidon, Norval) 30–60 mg daily has attracted the term 'tetracyclic': this drug may cause drowsiness but it too seems to be safer, in particular being relatively free from both cardiotoxic effects and anticholinergic side effects (dry mouth, constipation, etc).

Viloxazine (Vivalan) has the advantage of being virtually free of anticholinergic side effects but in the usual dose range (150–400 mg daily) does produce nausea in a proportion of patients. Its chemical structure is radically different from the other compounds.

These three drugs offer the prospect of profiles of therapeutic activity that may be quite distinct from those of the established drugs.

Monoamine oxidase inhibitors

The other important group of antidepressants are the **mono-amine oxidase inhibitors** (MAOIs).

In the central nervous system impulses are conveyed from one neuron to the next by means of chemical transmitters (amines) which include noradrenaline and 5-hydroxytryptamine (5HT; serotonin). The stimulation is more intense if the amount of amine present is increased. Normally, the amine disappears from the nerve junction:

(a) Through re-uptake back into the nerve cells from which they were released.

(b) Through destruction by the enzyme monoamine oxidase.

The tricyclic antidepressants block method (a) and the MAOIs block method (b), thus indirectly increasing cerebral amines.

The chemistry of the MAOIs is related to isoniazid, a drug used in treating tuberculosis. The first MAOI introduced was iproniazide (Marsilid). It was found to be hepatotoxic and is no longer used. There are two chemical groups of MAOIs:

1 Non-hydrazines, e.g. tranylcypromine (Parnate). It is rarely used because it is hepatotoxic and also seems to produce a hypertensive crisis more readily than the following drugs.

2 Hydrazines. The most frequently used are phenelzine (Nardil) 15–60 mg daily, isocarboxazide (Marplan) 10–40 mg daily, and nialamide (Niamid) 25–100 mg daily.

The MAOIs are chiefly used for treating depressive neurosis and phobic anxiety states. In the latter instance they are usually combined with a benzodiazepine. They are used particularly in depression unresponsive to tricyclic antidepressants. Although many psychiatrists dispute their usefulness, in many instances they do seem to be effective and dramatic in their antidepressant action.

MAOIs take 7–10 days to exert a therapeutic effect, and if effective, should be given for 12 weeks or more.

Their **principal side effects** are postural hypotension, ataxia, drowsiness, a dry mouth, difficulty with micturition, loss of sexual potency, insomnia, jaundice and constipation.

If combined with **tyramine** or catecholamines a hypertensive crisis may occur. Subarachnoid haemorrhage may develop if a congenital (berry) cerebral aneurysm is present.

Accordingly, all patients on MAOIs are advised to avoid **tyramine rich foods,** e.g. cheese, yoghurt, chocolate, Marmite, Bovril, other yeast extracts, bananas, broad beans, Chianti and heavy beers.

Hypertensive crisis sometimes occur if the patient is taking methyldopa (an antihypertensive drug) or tricyclic antidepressants at the same time. The few tricyclic antidepressants that are currently thought to be relatively safe with MAOIs include trimipramine and amitryptiline.

MAOIs potentiate alcohol, morphia and pethidine.

Since sympathomimetic (adrenaline-like) drugs are present in remedies for coughs and colds that are sold over the counter in drug stores and chemists' shops, patients are advised to take no drugs or medicines without consulting their doctor.

L-tryptophan

The current theory is that both tricyclics and MAOIs work by increasing available amounts of neurotransmitters in the brain. The transmitters include not only catecholamines (e.g. noradrenaline) but also indoleamines such as 5-hydroxytryptamine (5HT, serotonin).

Since L-tryptophan is a precursor of 5HT this drug has been tried for the same purpose.

Although its effectiveness as an antidepressant has not been established conclusively, L-tryptophan hes been used with some degree of success **in cases of resistant depression,** i.e. depression which is unresponsive to MAOIs, tricyclics, or ECT.

In these cases L-tryptophan is combined with an MAOI for a period of 3 to 6 weeks.

Furthermore, it is a very attractive drug because, being a natural constituent of the diet, it is virtually non-toxic. It is available as Pacitron or, in combination with vitamins, as Optimax. The recommended dose range is 3 g to 6 g daily.

Drowsiness is the most common side effect.

Lithium salts

Lithium salts have become an accepted treatment for the prevention of recurrence of manic depressive illness. They are probably more effective in controlling the frequency and severity of mania and hypomania rather than depression.

Lithium is given in oral tablet form as lithium carbonate (Camcolit) or in a slow release form (Priadel).

The precise mode of action is not known but intracellular replacement of sodium by lithium does occur. The dose is adjusted until the plasma lithium level is between 0.5–1.5 mmol/l. Toxic effects occur when the serum level rises above 2.0 mmol/l.

The more important side effects are fine tremor of the fingers and unsteadiness, nausea, vomiting, diarrhoea, lethargy and polyuria.

A large overdose produces coarse limb tremor, athetoid movements, confusion, stupor and convulsions. Long term usage sometimes produces a non-toxic goitre and hypothyroidism.

Patients are kept on lithium indefinitely and careful assessment is therefore required before using this drug. It is contraindicated in renal disease, hypertension and in pregnancy.

Miscellaneous drug treatments

Propranolol (30–200 mg daily) is a beta-adrenergic blocking agent. It relieves symptoms due to excessive adrenaline release (e.g. tachycardia, palpitations and probably tremor).

It has been used in the treatment of phobic anxiety and anxiety states, with some effect, but it is still in an experimental stage.

It is contraindicated in asthmatics and during pregnancy.

Antabuse (disulfiram) and **Abstem** (citrated calcium carbimide) are used in the treatment of chronic alcohol dependence. They interfere with the metabolism of alcohol, allowing acetaldehyde to accumulate in the blood.

If a patient on a maintenance dose of either drug ingests alcohol, a sequence of severely unpleasant symptoms occurs, acting as a deterrent to further drinking. For example, tightness of the chest, shortness of breath, generalized vasodilatation and a drop in blood pressure, faintness and tachycardia. Nausea, vomiting and collapse may also occur.

The dosage of Antabuse is 400–800 mg daily and of Abstem 100–400 mg daily.

Vitamins

Vitamins of the B group play an essential part in carbohydrate metabolism and nerve cells depend on carbohydrate metabolism for their energy requirements.

Vitamin B deficiencies are nearly always multiple and some result in psychiatric illness, for example, the confusional states in vitamin B_1 (aneurine or thiamine) deficiency (beriberi), and vitamin B_2 deficiency (pellagra) and the mental disorders found in chronic alcoholism. Individuals with anorexia or depression who eat little develop secondary vitamin deficiencies.

All these conditions are treated with high potency preparations of mixed B vitamins orally or by intramuscular injection. For example, Parentrovite, a standard preparation, is given I.M. 10 ml daily for 6–7 days.

Intellectual impairment sometimes accompanied by depression and paranoid features often occurs in vitamin B_{12} deficiency (e.g. with pernicious anaemia). It is treated with daily injections of vitamin B_{12} (cyanocobalamin) $1000 \mu g$ daily for 10 days and by regular injections subsequently.

Electroconvulsive therapy (ECT, electroplexy)

ECT was first used in the 1930s by a Hungarian psychiatrist, von Meduna, in the mistaken belief that schizophrenia and epilepsy were biologically antagonistic – that is, he believed that the induction of a fit would ameliorate schizophrenia. The precise mechanism of action is still not known.

Epileptic fits were at one time induced by the intravenous injection of cardiazol and the intramuscular injection of camphor. Both were found to be dangerous and in 1937 an electric shock was first used by Cerletti in Italy.

Inducing an unmodified electric shock resulted in many complications, especially fractures or dislocations of the spinal vertebrae and limb bones or joints, and damage to the teeth and tongue.

The introduction of a muscle relaxant and an anaesthetic before giving the shock was a major advance in the 1950s. This **'modified'** **ECT** eliminated most complications and also the unpleasantness of being awake yet totally paralysed.

The technique of ECT

Patients should always be told about the recommendation to give them ECT, their consent obtained, and the treatment explained so as to reassure them.

A routine physical examination is done, as in any case when an anaesthetic is to be given, and food and drink omitted for 4–6 hours prior to the treatment. The bladder is emptied and false teeth removed.

Anaesthesia is induced with a short acting intravenous barbiturate (e.g. sodium pentothal or methohexitone). As soon as sleep is induced, a muscle relaxant is given intravenously, such as succinylcholine 20–70 mg according to weight or previous response. The total muscle relaxation produced is preceded by involuntary twitching (fasciculation) of facial and limb muscles due to depolarization.

The patient is then insufflated with oxygen using a face mask and breathing bag and a rubber gag put between the teeth.

A standard ECT machine (e.g. the 'Ectron') is used to administer the current. Two electrodes, soaked in a 30% saline or bicarbonate solution are placed over the fronto-temporal area of the skull, and a current of 110 V (volts) passed between the electrodes for 0.5–2.0 s (seconds). A modified grand mal seizure is produced. If muscle relaxation is profound, the only evidence of the seizure is slight twitching of the ocular or facial muscles.

If a convulsion fails to occur, the procedure may be repeated once more. Further attempts on the same occasion would tend to produce excessive amnesia and confusion.

After the seizure has subsided, an airway is inserted and the patient again oxygenated. He is then turned on his left side and kept under nursing observation until full consciousness is recovered 5–10 minutes later.

The treatment is given two or three times weekly. An average course of treatment is 6–8 ECT.

The physical contraindications for treatment are:

1 A history of severe ischaemic heart disease, heart failure or a recent myocardial infarct.
2 A current chest infection.
3 Organic brain disease, for example a cerebral tumour (which sometimes presents as depression).
4 Depersonalization symptoms with which patients often become worse after ECT.

None of the above are absolute contraindications, and each must be weighed on its own merits.

Pregnancy and old age are not contraindications.

The indications for treatment are:

1 Severe depression, either unresponsive to antidepressant drugs, or where there is pressing urgency (e.g. because of suicidal tendencies). For example:

(a) The depressive phase of manic depressive psychosis, and other endogenous depressions.
(b) Reactive depression, especially when it has developed psychotic features.
(c) Puerperal depression.
(d) Depression in the involutional period of life.

As in the case of antidepressant drugs, ECT is more likely to prove effective when the patient is over 40 years of age and where the clinical picture includes early morning wakening and weight loss.
2 In mania and hypomania if treatment with drugs does not act soon enough.
3 In schizophrenia resistant to drug treatment, especially when an affective component is present, for example, agitation, excitement or depression, as in schizoaffective states, catatonic schizophrenia and some paranoid states.
4 More rarely, to terminate an organic confusional state.
ECT is a safe treatment. (Death occurred in only one case out of 28 000 cases in a recent study.)

The complications of ECT are:

1 Slight amnesia for remote and recent events, which may last several weeks, especially in patients given too many treatments over too short a period of time.
2 Mild disorientation, especially in the senile or arteriosclerotic patient.
3 Excessive or frequent use of ECT over a prolonged period of time has been thought to result in minimal permanent brain damage.
4 Fractures and dislocations, which are very rare if 'modified' ECT is used.
5 Occasionally mild feelings of unreality lasting for one or two weeks after treatment.

Unilateral ECT is associated with few side effects, and especially less amnesia. It is standard practice with many psychiatrists. Both electrodes are placed on the same side of the head (over the frontal and mastoid areas) on the non-dominant side, that is, on the right side in right handed people and vice versa.

Continuous narcosis

This is a useful treatment for patients with acute anxiety tension states or phobic anxiety, especially if the individual is restless, uncooperative, aggressive or hysterical in his behaviour.

The technique aims at inducing 12–18 hours of sleep in each 24 hour period, adjusted so that the patient is able to feed comfortably and attend to elimination of the faeces and urine. He must also be exercised briefly several times daily.

Narcosis is induced with a mixture of drugs:

1 Amylobarbitone sodium, 1–200 mg 6 hourly (oral dose) in combination with
2 Diazepam, 5–15 mg 6 hourly (oral dose).
3 If necessary, chlorpromazine may be used as a substitute or added in combination in doses of 50–100 mg 6 hourly (oral dose).

At times, it may be necessary to give one or other of these drugs intramuscularly.

The drugs are slowly tapered off after 5–10 days. During the narcosis, fluid and food intake should be measured and the patient's general physical condition, blood pressure, pulse rate, temperature and urine output monitored. The urine is tested daily for ketones.

This form of treatment must be used with great caution because of the possible serious complications of narcosis – e.g. inhalation pneumonia and electrolyte imbalance.

Insulin coma therapy is no longer used because of its proven lack of specific effect and its potential dangerousness. It used to be a standard treatment for schizophrenia until the 1950s. In the treatment, increasingly large doses of insulin were given daily to produce hypoglycaemic coma each day for 40–50 days.

Modified insulin therapy is also infrequently used. Its use is reserved for a minority of patients with intractable anxiety tension states or chronic depression who have anorexia and **progressive severe weight loss**. It is sometimes used in patients with anorexia nervosa. Patients are treated in hospital and given small but increasing daily doses of insulin (for example, 10 units insulin initially working up to 70–80 units daily over a period of 10–20 days). The injection of insulin produces mild hypoglycaemic symptoms, such as hunger, palpitations, sweating and restlessness. An hour after the injection has been given, the patient is fed with a high carbohydrate meal and heavily sugared drinks. 0.5–1 kg daily weight increase usually occurs.

If severe hypoglycaemia occurs during treatment it is rectified by administering a glucose solution via a stomach tube or i.v. injection of glucose or i.m. glucagon.

Abreactive techniques

Abreactive techniques are used in three situations:

1   In mute or amnesic patients.
2   In individuals too anxious or embarrassed to be able to discuss emotionally stressful events.
3   In individuals who have suppressed recent traumatic emotional experiences and the feelings associated with them, with the consequent production of psychological symptoms, for example hysterical conversion symptoms such as amnesia, paralysis of limbs or blindness, or the **depersonalization syndrome**, in which the patient feels the surroundings to be unreal (derealization) and his own body to be strange (depersonalization).

In the first two instances, **narcoanalysis** is attempted. The patient is given a small dose of intravenous barbiturate (5% sodium amylobarbitone or 25% sodium pentothal or methohexitone) slowly over a period of 10–30 minutes.

Mild clouding of consciousness, drowsiness, relief of tension, relaxation and disinhibition are produced, and the patient is allowed to talk about his problems.

In the third situation, **abreaction** is attempted. The patient is encouraged to relive and recount the suppressed traumatic experience. Strong suggestions may be made simultaneously.

The recollection and discussion of formerly 'forgotten' or unconscious emotional events results in a highly charged emotional state in which the patient, whilst reliving the experience, becomes restless, tearful, angry or relieved.

The abreaction situation process itself may sometimes be therapeutic, and it is not always necessary for specific traumatic events to be remembered.

Methylamphetamine (10–30 mg i.v. in 20 ml saline) is sometimes used with an i.v. barbiturate or by itself, to produce a more pronounced abreaction.

Other methods of abreaction less commonly used are the inhalation of **ether, nitrous oxide**, or a **carbon dioxide/oxygen mixture**. The use of these inhalants produces a more violent and dramatic abreaction.

Hypnosis produces, as with the abreactive agents, a state of heightened suggestibility during which the patient is more receptive to discussion of previous emotional experience, or its abreaction. The subject may be receptive to post hypnotic suggestion.

Patients do not show the EEG changes of sleep during hypnosis and usually remain in contact with part of their environment.

Hypnosis is frequently used to induce painless childbirth, in dental anaesthesia, and in the treatment of psychosomatic illness (for example, psychogenic asthma) and for the symptomatic relief of prolonged painful illness. It is time-consuming, and not of wide applicability to the majority of mental illnesses.

Psychosurgery

The most common operations are one or other variety of **leucotomy**.

The principle of all leucotomy procedures is to cut the white fibre tracts between the frontal lobe and the thalamus and hypothalamus. This pathway is responsible for the regulation of emotional responses and 'tension'.

The first operation was performed in 1936. In the original **standard pre-frontal leucotomy**, fibres were cut blindly using a needle like blunt instrument inserted into the brain through burr holes on each side of the skull near the coronal sutures.

After enormous numbers of operations had been done all over the world in an attempt at relieving the symptoms of schizophrenia and chronic depression, the operation fell into disrepute in the 1950s because of the high incidence of serious side effects.

The side effects (known as the **post leucotomy syndrome**) are:

1   Apathy, inertia and loss of initiative and drive.
2   Emotional flatness or slight euphoria.
3   Loss of judgement and coarsening of social behaviour.
4   Epileptic seizures.
5   Many patients become incontinent and 'vegetable-like'.

These effects were the result of a too extensive operation or because too much brain tissue was destroyed by haemorrhage at the time of operation.

In the 1960s, newer operations were developed with a more acceptable incidence of complications. They were of two types:

1   Modified leucotomy (either bimedial or rostral) – performed blindly through burr holes.
2   Bimedial orbital undercutting (where burr holes are made just above the frontal sinus and the area visualized at open operation).

In these operations, the aim is to cut a limited number of fibres in the lower medial quadrant of the frontal lobe.

In the 1970s, **stereotactic leucotomy** became popular. In this procedure, small areas of brain tissue are destroyed with great accuracy at a specific site, located by a complex method of three dimensional geometry using a special instrument after visualizing the air filled brain. The lesion is made by injecting alcohol, cryosurgery (freezing), electrical cauterization or implanting pellets of radioactive yttrium. If necessary, the lesion can be made larger.

Leucotomy should never be contemplated until other relevant forms of treatment have been extensively tried, usually for a period of several years.

The decision to operate is usually made after a conference involving patient, relatives, doctors, nurses, social workers and general practitioner.

Adequate rehabilitation and aftercare is essential, and the aim is to preserve intellectual function and minimize side effects at operation.

The indications for operation are:

1 Severe incapacitating obsessional, depressive or phobic illness.
2 Chronic incapacitating tension and anxiety.
3 Intractable severe pain.
4 A small number of schizophrenics uncontrollable with drugs.
5 The precise diagnosis is often unimportant and the presence of chronic anxiety, tension and subjective mental suffering, with or without delusions may be used as the indication for operation.

Patients who are relatively well adjusted personalities prior to operation, especially if they are conscientious and have a fair degree of 'drive' and initiative do best postoperatively.

Symptoms do not always disappear after operation: sometimes the patient may be less concerned and able to function more effectively in his life situation.

Psychopathic individuals and alcoholics do badly because their personality deficits may be exaggerated, and their difficulty in controlling their impulses made worse.

The operation is contraindicated if dementia or severe hypertension is present.

The mortality is 1–3%.

Other (rarer) operations performed are:

1 Cingulectomy (in severe obsessionals).
2 Amygdalotomy and thalamotomy (in aggressive, violent individuals).
3 Temporal lobectomy (in drug resistant epileptics and aggressiveness when a focal temporal lobe abnormality is demonstrable).

18 Behaviour Therapy

Behaviour therapy has become such an important and expanding part of psychiatric treatment that it requires discussion in some detail. It is important too, because it is a treatment that is being increasingly entrusted to paramedical staff – psychologists, nurses and occupational therapists.

The fundamental principle of behaviour therapy is that neuroses can be seen as learned patterns of maladaptive or inappropriate behaviour which are associated with anxiety. Constant repetition of the behaviour **reinforces** the maladaptive pattern (see pp. 84–86 for basic description).

Although the behaviour is usually learned in childhood, traumatic conditioning can occur at any age.

It is important to appreciate that the assumption that most behaviour is learned, and that the abnormal or neurotic symptoms can be modified or removed, **is not necessarily true**.

Behaviour therapy is used in the treatment of:

1   Anxiety, phobic and tension states.
2   Obsessional compulsive neuroses.
3   Sexual problems (impotence, frigidity and sexual deviations).
4   The correction of antisocial behaviour.
5   The retraining of patients with longstanding psychotic illness towards better socialization.

There are **two basic types of behaviour therapy:**

1   Classical conditioning therapy – where the response to the stimulus occurs inevitably.
2   Operant conditioning therapy – where the outcome depends on a voluntary act made by the patient.

159

1   Classical conditioning therapy

Unlearned behaviour is used to eliminate or modify unwanted behaviour. That is, he is conditioned to respond in a new way that is incompatible with his neurotic pattern. Three techniques are available:

(i)   Counterconditioning
(ii)   Positive reconditioning
(iii) Experimental extinction

(i)   Counterconditioning

Examples of this technique are:
(a)   Reciprocal inhibition with desensitization in imagination or practice.
(b)   Aversive conditioning.

(a)   Reciprocal inhibition depends on the principle that if a response which inhibits anxiety can be made to occur in the presence of an anxiety provoking stimulus, the **bond between the stimulus and anxiety will be weakened.**

The response used to inhibit anxiety (i.e. counterconditioning) is **deep muscular relaxation** and patients are trained progressively to relax mentally and physically.

A list of situations – 'the hierarchy' – is then constructed, ranging from events which provoke mild anxiety to those provoking severe anxiety. The patient, having been relaxed, is then asked to imagine and describe the **mildest** anxiety provoking situation **without** developing anxiety; the next and subsequent situations in the hierarchy are similarly dealt with. He then becomes **fully desensitized in imagination.**

The next step is to work progressively through the equivalent real life situation in order, again utilizing the relaxation procedure, i.e. **desensitization in practice**. For example: an agoraphobic patient might be accompanied by a nurse on short, then progressively longer walks from home, then allowed to do it alone in a graduated way.

The relaxation procedure can be rapidly enhanced by using IV methohexitone (a short acting barbiturate). 10–30 sessions of treatment are usually required. The procedure is often combined with **assertive training**, that is, learning to cope better by self assertion and expression in social situations that usually render the vulnerable or inadequate patient diffident and unsure, and the practice of assertive acts (behaviour rehearsal).

(b) Aversive conditioning. Here, the patient is presented (or punished) with an unpleasant stimulus, e.g. an electric shock or drug induced nausea and vomiting when he behaves in an undesirable way.

The behaviour and the stimulus are coupled together and arranged so that progressive reduction of the unwanted behaviour progressively removes the unpleasant stimulus. For example, in alcoholics, ingesting alcohol is associated with nausea and vomiting, produced by giving an injection of apomorphine a few minutes previously. Eventually, vomiting and nausea occur without the apomorphine; this results in distaste and fear when drinking is contemplated. This method has not proven to be of great benefit in the management of alcoholism.

(ii)   *Positive reconditioning*

This is used to treat nocturnal enuresis. A new motor habit is developed by awakening the patient with an alarm as soon as he excretes urine. The urine completes an electrical circuit in a specially designed mattress. The patient rapidly learns not to urinate in response to bladder stimulation during sleep.

(iii)   *Experimental extinction (negative practice)*

Here, an unwanted motor habit, e.g. facial tic or body movement is progressively weakened by repeated non-reinforcement (extinction) of the response (i.e. the tic). For example, the patient is made to repeatedly produce the tic for several hours and then relax, followed by further repeated sessions.

2   Operant conditioning therapies

These all aim at modifying or eliminating unwanted or inappropriate behaviour by providing rewards. Operant methods depend on a specific motor response from the patient. There are several varieties:

(i) Behaviour modification

In this form of operant conditioning a specific reward is provided when the inappropriate behaviour is corrected, and it is repeatedly reinforced over a period of days or weeks. It is chiefly used in the retraining of chronic patients in mental hospitals (especially chronic apathetic schizophrenics) and sociopathic personalities in prisons. The term **token economy** is often used for this type of treatment. That is, a gift or token is given as a reward after inappropriate behaviour has been corrected.

(ii) Social imitation and modelling

This method allows a patient to imitate the behaviour of a therapist he respects and trusts, thus reducing associated anxiety and altering unwanted behavioural patterns. Modelling and assertive training (social skills training) are often best practised in groups.

Other behaviour therapies

Other methods of behaviour therapy used in certain circumstances are:

Implosion (flooding)

This is virtually the opposite of conditioning. It is used in the treatment of specific phobias.

The patient is repeatedly exposed to the feared object or situation over an extended period of time – hours or even days, until his anxiety diminishes. It may be done in imagination, and then later in reality.

Response prevention (apotreptic) therapy

Here, the patient is actively prevented from performing the unwanted behaviour – which is usually a tedious obsessive compulsive ritual.

It must be remembered that although behaviour therapy is, in selected cases, remarkably effective, that:

1   It aims at removing symptoms rather than causes.
2   It is, therefore, best used in monosymptomatic conditions rather than complex neuroses.

3 Symptom substitution sometimes occurs, that is, removal of one symptom results in replacement by another, especially if the fundamental problems have not been adequately dealt with.

4 There are many similarities between behaviour therapy and other forms of psychotherapy and the effect of transference and suggestibility in behaviour therapy may be very important.

19 Psychotherapy

The term **psychotherapy** includes those forms of treatment that rely largely on talking with the patient (rather than on physical means such as drugs or ECT). There are three main aims of psychotherapy:

(a)   To reduce anxiety and distress to tolerable levels.

(b)   To improve patterns of behaviour so that the individual's actions are the most appropriate and best adapted to his circumstances.

(c)   To increase the patient's insight and awareness of his own feelings and reactions.

Many professionals (doctors, nurses, social workers etc.) try to achieve all these aims with an individual patient, and the techniques they use are complex. To make the methods clearer, however, we shall deal with each of these objectives in turn.

Anxiety reducing methods of psychotherapy

This group of techniques comes nearest to the way you naturally try to help friends and relatives when they are in trouble, and it includes sympathy, reassurance, advice and encouragement. However, you have to modify the approach for patients who are very distressed or disturbed. Bear in mind that under these circumstances patients find it difficult to relate to or get on with other people – their interpersonal relationships are impaired – and this means that they will find it more difficult to get on with **you**. They may find it difficult to accept your sympathy or to trust you. They are likely to be concerned with the idea that you are telling them what to do or 'pushing them around'. For the duration of their mental illness, at least, they are prone to feel not only guilty or low in self-esteem, but also to be critical of you and others, suspicious and irritable.

Because they may find it difficult to accept your help, you should offer it initially in a way that does **not demand a response from**

them. For instance, if you want to show sympathy, do not tell them how sorry you are for them in a way that makes them feel obliged to say 'thank you' or 'that's kind of you'. Make your remarks in low key, rather than being effusive or gushing. Often it is enough to say something like 'You must find it difficult to bear that'. Smiling brightly at the patient may result in him becoming embarrassed or guilty at not feeling like smiling back. By all means do offer sympathy if you feel it will comfort the patient, but gauge carefully the extent to which he can take it.

You have to be just as cautious with other **supportive** measures (as anxiety reducing techniques are often called). Obviously we would like to make the patient feel better by *reassuring* him. Remember that he may not be impressed if you say 'Don't worry, you'll be all right soon'. To begin with, if he is depressed it may be difficult to get him to see any hope in the future. Secondly, **allowing** yourself to be reassured by someone else involves putting your trust in him – something that is difficult for psychiatric patients. Again it is a question of making a demand on the patient that he feels unable to meet. Sometimes you can make this point explicit by saying 'I am sure you will feel a lot better in a few weeks time, but don't worry if you can't believe that at the moment'.

We should be careful not to give the patient spurious reassurance. If he says 'Will I be able to go home by the end of the week' pleadingly, it is too easy to say comfortingly 'Yes, yes, of course', so as to allay his intolerable anxiety. At the end of the week, when he is not quite ready for going home, he may well remember how you gave him false hope, and hold it against you. Your relationship with him is more important than a temporary lull in his fretting, and it would have been better at the time to have said something like 'I think you will be feeling a lot better by the end of the week' knowing that you have not really told him what he wants to hear.

Advice is fraught with difficulties even when it is given to persons who are in a serene frame of mind. You will need to know someone incredibly well before telling them who to marry. Whether he does well at a particular job depends on all sorts of value judgements, prejudices and deeply felt needs, and any one of these attitudes may be crucial to success or failure. Of course what you can do is ask him if he has **considered** a particular line of action and then, if it appeals, he can benefit from your suggestion: if it repels he will ignore it. When people are distressed and lacking in confidence, however, they are often their own worst enemies. When you make a positive suggestion, they may act on it and then afterwards say to you 'There you are, it all went wrong, it's your fault'. When you are tempted to make a suggestion first of all ask yourself, if it is so obviously what the patient should do, why he has not thought of it himself? Often there is an important obstacle to success that is not obvious at first sight – possibly even one that the patient is aware of. If after discussing the possibility it still seems the right thing to do, allow the patient to make the decision himself. Ask him if he feels that he can cope with the task. If he assures **you** that he can cope and make a go of it, he is far more likely to make the necessary effort than if you have assured **him** he can do it.

We have so far considered three supportive techniques – sympathy, reassurance and advice. There are many others that will occur to you in your day to day work – including encouragement, warmth, praise, comfort, companionship, understanding and respect. The same principles apply to each of them as did to the first three. They are all appropriate techniques to use at times, but should be used cautiously, and with a keen sensitivity towards the response of the patient to them. The important consideration is that it should make the patient feel better, not just make you feel better because you are doing something. Even experienced therapists have to beware of this trap.

We shall consider just one more supportive technique in detail since it is a little different from the others, and that is the technique of **suggestion**. By this we do not mean advice or counselling. It is well known that if a doctor gives a patient an injection for severe pain, that the pain may clear up dramatically in a few seconds even though the syringe contained nothing stronger than sterile water. This **placebo** effect, as it is called, can operate with tablets and capsules as well, and is a powerful force. The patient is convinced that his pain will improve, and that conviction is sufficient to alter his perception of the pain.

This is an example of **suggestion** in the sense that we are using it here. The doctor **suggests** that the patient will improve; if the patient believes him, then the chances are that he will feel better even if nothing else changes. One of the most extreme forms of suggestion is **hypnosis**. The hypnotist **suggests** to the subject that he is relaxing, having asked him previously to lie down. He suggests, perhaps, that his eyelids feel tired, having previously asked him to gaze hard at an object above his usual line of vision. By progressive suggestions the susceptible subject can go into a trance where his arm will feel light and rise up into the air if the hypnotist suggests it, or where he feels no pain if he is told he will not.

Hypnosis is an interesting technique, and it can be used to minimize or avoid the pain of dental extraction, childbirth or surgical operations. It has not so far proved to be of widespread value in psychiatry, but it is used in a method of treatment called **abreaction**. If a patient's mental illness follows a sudden frightening episode then sometimes he can be treated successfully by taking him back in memory to the incident and getting him to relive it in his mind's eye, going through (abreacting) all the emotional turmoil that was in some way blocked originally. To get a patient into the frame of mind where he is prepared to relive the episode various drugs can be injected intravenously (paradoxically stimulants as well as sedatives) or the technique of hypnosis can be used. These cases are not very common, however, outside wartime or major disasters (see pp. 155–156).

Behavioural psychotherapy (see pp. 159–163)

Behaviour therapy treats symptoms as abnormal conditioned reflexes. Let us suppose that a patient has a spider phobia. This means that not only does he have the fear of spiders that is present in many children and some adults, but that it is of a degree of severity that is enough to impair his life in some way by restricting his activities.

The behaviour therapist argues that developing a fear of spiders is a conditioned response. In the case of poisonous spiders this would have some biological advantage, but in the example described above the process has got out of hand, and has generalized to all spiders. The therapist takes the hypothetical view that if you can be **conditioned** to a pattern of behaviour, then you can be deconditioned. A scientific study of conditioned responses has shown many factors that influence their 'learning' and also how they can be extinguished – a body of knowledge known as **learning theory**.

One method of dealing with symptoms on these lines is called **desensitization**. For example the patient might be asked to imagine a spider 10 miles away; in his mind's eye he is asked to imagine it gradually nearer. The stimuli are increased in intensity over the treatment sessions, progressing through a **hierarchy** of feared situations. With successful treatment the patient ends up being able to handle (non-poisonous!) spiders with ease. The important proviso with this method is that the patient is not moved on to the more feared situation until he can handle the previous situation without distress. Various **supportive** measures may be used to enable him to achieve this progress, but it can be seen that no attempt is made to improve his understanding of how he developed the symptom in the first place, nor how it relates to the rest of his personality make up. The proof of the pudding is in the eating, and if the patient is satisfied at the end of his treatment in the sense that he is able to cope with his particular phobia without becoming unduly anxious, then such understanding and enlightenment about his character and mentality may be regarded as unnecessary frills and luxuries.

Insight-oriented psychotherapy

What for one patient is an unnecessary luxury is for another patient the very essence of treatment. Insight-oriented (or orientated) psychotherapy includes those forms of treatment that allow the patient to get in touch with his underlying feelings, with funda-mental parts of the mind that he is not normally aware of. For this reason it is sometimes called **depth** psychology. The most exten-sive version is known as **psychoanalysis**. In this form of treatment the patient lies on a couch, telling whatever thoughts that enter his mind, no matter how shocking or trivial ('free association'), while the analyst – who is mainly silent in the background – responds from time to time by making **interpretations**. These are state-ments about the unconscious reasons that the patient has for behaving the way he does. Since the patient has until then been unaware of his motivation, he may react with incredulity or denial. Alternatively he may feel helped and liberated by his under-standing. If the former feelings of antagonism prevail, he might find it difficult to talk – a feature that the analyst will identify as **resistance**.

You can see that the process of analysis itself can be one of emotional turmoil – sometimes an intense and painful one. So while the analyst starts his treatment armed with little more than the patient's voluntary utterances and uncorroborated assertions, gradually he can see for himself how the patient reacts.

The analyst is on the look-out for those slightly irrational or persistent expectations that we all have of other people's behaviour towards ourselves. For example some young men always expect women to be critical and wounding in their remarks. It may well be the case that this is because their own mothers have behaved in this way towards them. If these expectations influence or dominate their attitude towards every new female that they meet, then they are likely to experience problems in these relationships. Such a man, being ready to see remarks made by his new girlfriend as cutting, deflating or nagging, will find meeting women a painful experience, and similarly women will find his attitudes and assumptions irritating and tension producing.

We can now see that in the emotional relationships that the patient develops **towards his analyst** the unrealistic parts of his expectations may carry over with them echoes of earlier interpersonal experiences that he has had (starting with his parents). This unwitting transfer of previous attitudes so characterizes the intense feelings that the patient comes to have towards his analyst that this process is known as the **transference**. Over the three years or more that the analysis goes on for, this transference becomes more and more the material on which the skill of the analyst works, in a technique referred to as **analysis of the transference**.

In a full analysis the patient will have treatment sessions, each lasting 50 minutes, five days a week. Less intense forms of treatment along these lines are called psychoanalytically oriented psychotherapy.

In **group therapy** typically from eight to twelve patients assemble with the therapist (and possibly a trainee observer or a co-therapist). Ideally the conversational interchanges should crisscross from one member of the group to another, and often members of the group will be able to help each other with interpretations, without relying too heavily on the therapist. **Resistance** takes forms that may be different from those found in individual treatment. For instance, pairing, in which two group members dominate the discussion by addressing all their remarks to each other, effectively prevents the group as a whole from carrying out its work, and can 'protect' the pair concerned from insights offered by others.

Group therapy is not just a cheap way of treating twelve people. It is valuable for those patients who would not accept interpretations from an individual therapist. You cannot say to yourself 'He's just trying to prove a theory' or 'He's got a bee in his bonnet about obsessional character traits' of your therapist if in fact the interpretations are being made by all your fellow group members. It is also valuable for those individuals who need to see living examples (acted out in front of them) of their own interpersonal problems.

Other forms of psychotherapy

In some ways supportive (anxiety reducing) psychotherapy (as described earlier) and typical analytical (insight-oriented) psycho-therapy are at opposite poles. There are many forms of treatment that come somewhere in between. If you were allowed to listen to a psychotherapeutic session you might have a lot of trouble telling which school the therapist belonged to. To begin with the chances are that the patient would be doing most of the talking. In most forms of psychotherapy great value is placed on **listening to** the patient. Suppose that you wait until the patient at last stops talking, what words of wisdom might you hear the therapist utter then? Probably something like 'Tell me some more about that' or a comment that in some other way encourages the patient to go on talking.

The therapist may occasionally go a little further and link up a few of the topics that the patient has covered, starting his remark with 'It seems to me that what you are saying is ...', keeping to what is being openly stated, and not trying to infer unconscious motives. This technique of reflecting back to the patient what he has been saying is sometimes called **clarification**. The patient generally agrees with the summing up, is probably pleased with the evidence that at least his therapist has been listening to him, and may be stimulated into further revelations.

Confrontation is a procedure that lies somewhere between the mild clarification on the one hand and the demanding interpretation on the other. The therapist collects together evidence that the **patient is behaving in a certain way** (e.g. an aggressive manner), presenting to the patient a description that may be unwelcome but that does not delve into the unconscious.

If you were to study psychotherapists at work you might find that they were spending 90 to 95% of their time using fairly neutral techniques like listening and clarification, so that only rarely did they need to make an intervention that was positively supportive or interpretative. It would seem that **listening** is therapeutic in itself. It is certainly an art worth cultivating.

20 Psychiatric Nursing

The functions of the psychiatric nurse have changed considerably in recent years. Some nurses have taken on quite new roles, such as behaviour therapist. More usually the nurse acts as part of a therapeutic team, where in addition to her traditional work she has the opportunity to accept an active part in other aspects of treatment such as occupational therapy and group therapy. Her work is less dominated by authority relationships, both in her dealings with other staff and in her dealings with patients.

A great strength of her position in the treatment team comes from the fact that she is with the patient throughout the day. What does she do during these long hours of patient contact?

With patients whose main disability is their distress and anxiety she will comfort them, sympathize, encourage and use a variety of approaches all designed to lower anxiety levels. These techniques are similar to those described in the section on psychotherapy (pp. 164–170), where you will also find some of the precautions you need to adopt when using them.

There are parallels between the nursing of the psychiatrically ill and nursing patients in pain and physical distress. There are, however, a number of differences. Some of the most important are:

(a) The extent to which symptoms of anxiety and depression rule the clinical picture with most psychiatric patients.

(b) The fact that these unpleasant emotions exceed what would be justified by the patient's environmental stresses.

(c) The lack of response of many psychiatric patients to ordinary reassurance.

(d) The impairment of human relationships that such patients often show – with lack of trust, suspicion and hostility.

(e) The fact that there are far fewer physical nursing procedures that the nurse can use to show her concern.

Her main task will not necessarily be finding words of comfort and reassurance but **listening**. A patient often derives a great deal of support from being able to ventilate his problems – getting it 'off his chest'. It is helpful for him to feel that someone else is concerned, and understands (even if incompletely) how he feels. The listening can be done silently without murmuring sympathies, and even while carrying out some manual task, as long as occasionally the nurse says something that shows that she has heard what was being said.

In this way the patient does most of the talking. When the nurse does say something, it will often be a question or statement designed to encourage the patient to continue talking. When she comments on the patient's utterances, as far as possible she will avoid criticism or rejection of the patient's moral values. This **non-judgemental attitude** is the hallmark of all mental health professional staff. It does not mean that you are not entitled to have your own private opinions and standards. It **does** mean that you do not impose them on the patient.

In this way she shows her respect for the patient as a person, who is entitled to his own religious, moral and political beliefs.

To make this clearer, consider what happens if the patient talks about clearly delusional beliefs. Let us say that he believes that he is the King of Ruritania. The correct response to this is neither to confirm nor deny his belief. It is certainly useless to deny it and try to argue him out of his conviction. Far from convincing him that you are right, you will merely show him, in his eyes, that you have failed to understand him. It is equally wrong to 'humour' him, in the sense of saying 'Yes, yes, of course you are the King of Ruritania'. Apart from the fact that he may only partly believe it himself (so that he thinks you are a fool for going along with him) it also, and more seriously, puts you into an intolerably false position. As far as you can you should keep your relationship with the patient one of honesty. Although, as we have seen, you do not blurt out every criticism and blunt statement that occurs to you, you should try to avoid making definitely untrue statements.

You may have to talk to him **about** his delusion. How can you avoid confirming or denying it then? Usually it is not too difficult. You do not talk to him about the **fact** that he is the king, you talk to him about his **belief** that he is the king. The same applies to delusions of ill-health. You may say 'I can see that you are very worried about the idea that you have cancer of the bowel'. It is easy to appreciate that there is an important distinction between saying this and saying 'I can see you are very worried about your cancer of the bowel'.

This approach can be considered as part of a general plan of **trying to keep the confidence of the patient in you**. A further illustration of this is the problem dealing with the suspicious patient. For instance, if you have to see the relatives of a patient, it is worth trying, whenever possible, to have the patient present at the interview. The obvious disadvantage is that the relatives may not feel so free to say unflattering things about the patient while he is present, and so you may lose some of the information that you would otherwise have obtained from them. Usually this is a small price to pay for the benefit of improved trust of the patient in you. He does not feel that you are 'going behind his back' and colluding with his relatives. A variant on this technique occurs, for instance, when you have to get in touch with his employers. The patient is likely to be very concerned about what you might say to them. You can help him here by allowing him to stay in the room while you make the call, starting the conversation with the statement that you are phoning about Mr Smith who you have in the room with you.

Violent patients

The idea of being attacked by a violent patient is probably one of the most frightening prospects of someone coming into contact with the mentally ill for the first time. After a while such anxieties are allayed when it can be seen that such incidents are fairly uncommon, and that when they occur they do not usually cause permanent physical harm to the staff concerned. Compared with the 'bedlam' image of the past, psychiatric wards have become fairly peaceful places since the advent of major tranquillizers.

Nevertheless the risk can be reduced even more by the use of the correct psychological approach. The aim should be to recognize the high risk patients and to act to prevent them getting into situations where they feel they have to act out their hostile feelings. We have just considered some ways, for instance, of helping patients feel less persecuted or paranoid. Further steps in this direction are to improve communications with mistrustful patients. They should be told exactly what is happening in their treatment programme, and in fact this should be repeated frequently in case they have not taken it in the first time. Even more important that the actual information that you give them is the atmosphere that you build up that conveys your obvious intention not to keep them in the dark nor to hold things back from them.

Try to be aware of how the patient sees **you**. For instance if you are worried about a particular patient, tension and anxiety may be revealed in your facial expression. The facial expression may be misinterpreted by the patient as one of **hostility** on your part. It is often helpful to reassure such patients by saying 'don't be frightened'. Apart from any reassuring effect that this statement has on the patient, it helps to remind you that fear is just what he may be experiencing, and helps to show him that you are concerned about his feelings.

This type of attitude and behaviour on your part can help defuse an otherwise explosive situation, so that the patient settles down once more. It should be obvious from the comments made above that the nurse can deal with situations like this more efficiently if she is calm, confident and reassuring. But how do you **get** to be calm and confident about these situations in the first place? Obviously experience with psychiatric patients is a very important factor: it is noticeable how patients that have proved impossible to handle elsewhere often settle down with apparently miraculous ease when they are transferred to a ward staffed by psychiatrically trained nurses.

Preaching the value of experience is not much help to the nurse who is just starting her psychiatric training, however. At this stage it can be very helpful if she has some practice sessions in which staff pretend to be violent patients, and various manoeuvres are tried. This helps partly because you find out about some of the physical steps you can take, and probably more because you are rehearsing an event that would otherwise be frightening by its unfamiliarity as well as by the inherent risk of damage to the person.

It also helps if the nurse understands that it is legitimate for her to use reasonable force in restraining an impulsive patient, and if she knows that her senior nursing colleagues and the medical staff will back her up in her judgement.

Suicidal patients

Violent behaviour carried out by the patient is much more likely to be against **himself** than against others. Suicidal thoughts are very common amongst people with mental disorder. Many patients get over this phase without any dramatic medical intervention, but if these ideas become dominant then it may be necessary to admit the patient to a psychiatric ward.

Such a patient feels hopeless. In his severe pessimism he sees no prospect of ever improving. The danger comes when a wave of desperation overwhelms him and he decides that he can put up with his painful feelings no longer. Although you may know that his judgement is false, and that in a week or two he will be feeling quite different, it is useless arguing with him about his depressive delusions or ideas.

In these circumstances admission to a psychiatric ward is often a great help in itself. The patient may have been dismayed at the idea to start with – among the many fears that patients have about being admitted as a patient are:

(a) The stigma of being labelled a psychiatric case ('What will people think?').
(b) The fear that he will lose his liberty ('Will I be locked up?').
(c) The fear of 'catching' insanity from other patients.
(d) The fear of violence from other patients.

Having been admitted, and seen that much of his fear is exaggerated, the patient usually feels some relief. Although with half of his mind he believes there is no hope for him, with the other half he feels that there is at least a chance that something can be done for him. Whatever the reasoning, it is usual to find, **provided they are not provoked,** that such patients are less inclined to act out their self-destructive urges just after admission.

Unless they are provoked? What I have in mind is putting the patient alone in a fifth floor room with the window open, or with a long sash cord dangling, or with a glass object to hand. Faced with this situation, the suicidal patient may come to the conclusion that the staff do not think he is seriously depressed, and then decide that since no one understands or cares he will show them how wrong they are and at the same time end his own suffering.

Care in the ward. Let us assume that we now have our suicidal patient in the ward. How should the staff cope with him? The first question is how far to go in removing dangerous objects from his person. This is a matter of judgement, and each ward has its own customs. The pros and cons are as follows. If you do **not** remove razor blades, sharp knives and similar objects then (a) the staff remain anxious in case the patient damages himself and (b) the patient may feel 'provoked', as described earlier.

A disadvantage of removing these articles is that the patient feels that he is in a very artificial and restrictive atmosphere which makes it difficult to form natural relationships with the staff.

Can it actually make suicide more likely to take away his razor blades? This is a possibility. In the section on psychotherapy we considered the effects of suggestion (pp. 166–167). The powers of suggestion can work for ill as well as for good. On the whole if a patient has not yet become depressed to the point of contemplating suicide, then you are not likely to 'put the idea into his head' either by removing knives or by asking him if he has suicidal feelings. If a patient is seriously suicidal already, though, then it is possible that he may form the opinion that you are taking away these objects because you **know** that he is fated to kill himself. He may then feel that he may as well end it all as soon as possible – and if a patient is really determined to kill himself it is very difficult to avoid him finding some way of at least making the attempt.

Here is a difficult dilemma. On the one hand you do not want him to feel (by leaving him in possession of dangerous articles) that you are not taking him seriously. On the other hand you do not want (by taking them away) to make him feel that you think his suicide is just a matter of time.

The skill of the nurse shows itself in solving this dilemma. If you decide that the best policy is to remove these articles, then it must be done carefully. You will point out that you are trying to help him in this way, just in case he gets an impulse to harm himself which he finds difficult to resist. With adequate explanation and tact most patients will take this procedure in the right spirit.

If, in a doubtful case, you are thinking about letting him keep such possessions, you may wish to bring him into the decision by asking him if he can cope with the responsibility of looking after them. If a patient gives a plain, straightforward opinion that he can deal with the situation, then you are probably safe. If he gives an uncertain reply then you will want to think again, and consider taking the articles until he feels sure that he can control his impulses.

If you think that the patient is hoarding drugs in his locker, it may be necessary to make a search. Whenever possible this should be done with his knowledge, and preferably when he is present.

Patients may try to take their own lives not just by physical methods but also by chemical means. Some save up their medication day by day until they consider that they have enough tablets with which to kill themselves. This is one reason why the nurse should always be aware of the possibility that the patient is not taking the tablets he is given. There are various other reasons why patients do not take their medicine, and this subterfuge is not confined to psychiatric wards (it was well known at one hospital that antenatal in-patients threw their iron tablets out of the window). Nevertheless on a psychiatric ward the nurse has to be particularly vigilant. In cases of doubt she should ask to see the patient swallow the tablet and then inspect his mouth to make sure that it does not remain secreted under the tongue or between gum and cheek. This is again a situation that calls for tact and discretion, but even in non-suicidal patients the deception may lead to weeks or months of unnecessary ill-health.

The disturbed patient

The term 'disturbed' is rather vague and can mean little more than severely ill in the mind. Some situations that might come into this category are dealt with elsewhere in the book. States of delirium (pp. 63–65) and dementia (pp. 70–72) come under organic brain disease. The problem of delusions was dealt with when considering paranoid states (pp. 172–173) and we have just discussed problems with violent or suicidal patients.

Psychotic patients may act in strange inappropriate ways that are difficult to understand. Depressed patients may sit about doing nothing for hours, or restlessly pace up and down. Hypomanic patients rush about with ceaseless energy, interfering and demanding. Other patients act out their problems by coming back to the ward drunk, taking illicit drugs, or acting in other socially unacceptable ways.

One of the main tasks of the nurse is to **be with** the patient. She has to be adaptable since it is clear that what is demanded of her varies from one situation to another. The behaviour of the schizophrenic patient is unpredictable. With him the nurse needs to be vigilant and alert for the unexpected move. Such patients are usually unable to deal with intense emotional relationships and often find it helpful if the staff themselves are fairly cool and unstimulating. The depressed patient should not be allowed to turn his face to the wall and give up life completely. His activity and socialization have to be encouraged in a gentle and gradual manner.

The hypomanic patient can be a great strain for the nursing staff. Left to himself, he may test all the rules to breaking point. If 'lights-out' is at 10 p.m. he will be up later. If confronted with this breach of regulations he will say 'But it is only a quarter past ten. Surely you are not that rigid?'. In this and similar ways he will put the staff in the wrong, making even the most liberal nurse appear to be authoritarian and arbitrary.

He may even set one member of staff against another. Hypomanic patients frequently seem to possess considerable skill in knowing what will flatter you, or what will really get 'under your skin' and irritate you. By flattering one member of staff such a patient may obtain privileges that have been denied by another. Under these circumstances it is crucial that the staff should discuss with each other (e.g. in group meetings) the appropriate management of the patient to reduce misunderstandings. Staff should recognize their own nettled feelings, and accept them as products of the patient's illness. It is necessary to set limits to the patient's behaviour and to stick to these agreed limits even if the patient does make you feel you are being unreasonable.

Acting out patients

Many patients are not able to accept the frustration of keeping their feelings to themselves, or merely talking about their problems. From time to time they yield to the urge to show their feelings dramatically in their behaviour. They break windows, walk out of group meetings or ward rounds, abscond from the hospital, take overdoses or break the rules (even in places where there are very few rules).

The staff have a conflict in trying to deal with this **acting out behaviour**. They can treat it understandingly and indulgently, when they run the risk of actually encouraging it: the patient may feel rewarded for his actions by getting sympathy and attention. Or they may treat it sternly and with discipline, by withdrawing privileges or in some way using sanctions to discourage such activities: then they run the risk of making the patient feel rejected and misunderstood, and losing any sense of trust.

Somehow the staff have to find a response that maintains the limits of acceptable behaviour but on the other hand keeps the goodwill of the patient. This situation is a great test of skill, and staff members will find many ways of solving this dilemma. Let us try to illustrate one way by looking at a common form of acting out – drinking. Many psychiatric wards have a rule that patients may not consume alcohol. Some of the reasons for such a restriction include the possibility of interaction with psychotropic drugs, the tantalizing effects on recovering alcoholics in the same ward, and the difficulty of giving psychological help to someone whose thinking is fuddled while drunk.

What do you do when a patient returns to the ward in an inebriated state? Pointing out the rules, and withdrawing permission for leaving the ward may not be the best responses. An alternative is to tell the patient that you see this lapse as a sign of his dissatisfaction with his progress. You take the line that he would not have been tempted to indulge unless he was suffering severe tension. You may also point out that it suggests that he is impatient with the attempts so far to relieve his tension. So far, then, you have taken his lapse seriously, and you have tried to show some understanding of what drove him to it.

The next thing is to ask him in future to tell someone when he feels like doing it again, so that other ways can be found of coping with these feelings. You may also ask him to try to exert more control himself over his behaviour.

If done properly this combination of responses will leave the patient in little doubt that you are trying to understand and help him, but that you take a serious view of the disruptive effect of his actions.

Being with the patient

Most of the time the average patient is not behaving in a dramatic way, so that violence, acting out, suicide or disturbed behaviour are just distant possibilities. A more frequent problem is that, far from being frantic or excited, the patient is rather apathetic, inert, passive and in need of encouragement to carry out even minor tasks. A stranger coming into a psychiatric ward may see it as quite a dull place.

The nurse therefore needs to be very adaptable, stimulating one patient and calming another. A good principle is to try to work with the **healthy** parts of the patient's mind. Almost all psychiatric patients can talk sensibly on some topics that interest them. So the nurse has to tr to encourage the patients to behave as normally as possible, yet bing constantly on the look-out for abnormal signs.

Her observations are recorded in the progress sheets or cards. These notes should be as informative as possible, pointing out to what degree the patient seems ill, to what degree he seems well, and what he is like now compared with previously. Since the nurse spends longer with the patient than any other member of staff these notes can be of the utmost value.

Frequently the nursing staff take responsibility for serving the meals to the patients. This has great symbolic importance, since nourishment and feeding are identified with help and sympathy. Other duties that may come the way of the nurse in some units include occupational therapy, behaviour therapy and group therapy.

The nurse is responsible for giving the patient his medication. During this procedure a sensitive nurse can learn a lot about the patient's attitudes. Reluctance by the patient to take his tablets should be carefully noted. It may indicate that the patient is not happy about his treatment in general.

Many patients who surreptitiously evade taking oral tablets improve dramatically when, for example, their psychotropic drugs are given by long acting injections.

A psychiatric nurse has to play different roles according to the setting. Her job in looking after demented psychogeriatric in-patients will contrast strongly with that of working in a therapeutic community run for adolescents. Other varied situations include the acute admission ward of a large psychiatric hospital, community work where patients are seen in their own homes, attachment to a long stay ward in a general hospital, administrative work supervising other nurses, and work in a day hospital or outpatient clinic.

21 The Organization of Psychiatric Care

In the UK, until the late 1950s, mental hospitals were isolated in their relationship to general hospitals. They were too large, essentially custodial, authoritarian, and operated on 'locked door' principles, so that patients had little freedom of movement, even within the hospital.

There was a rigid hierarchy and relationship between doctors, nurses and paramedical staff – social workers and occupational therapists.

Little stress was placed on group behaviour, constructive rehabilitation and community aftercare.

Changes in public attitudes, medical thinking, and the introduction of a new Mental Health Act in 1959 resulted in psychiatrists and nurses critically re-examining their role in respect of their traditional responsibilities. The NHS reorganization in 1974 provided further impetus for the imaginative development of psychiatric hospital care and after care in the community.

In the mental hospital setting, radical changes evolved. They coincided with revolutionary changes in psychopharmacology which have altered the natural history of depression (by the use of tricyclic and MAOI antidepressant drugs) and schizophrenia (by the use of phenothiazines and butyrophenones).

The role of the hospital superintendent was abolished and small **treatment teams**, led by a consultant psychiatrist (known as the responsible medical officer), plus a support staff of junior doctors, a psychologist, social workers, occupational therapists and nurses, were formed. Each team was allocated a **catchment area** in the community and attempts were made to bring psychiatric treatment and facilities **into the community** rather than concentrating on the hospital in isolation. (A catchment area is a geographical area in which all patients becoming mentally ill are dealt with by a specific consultant or appropriate psychiatric unit.)

In addition to these teams, attempts were made at altering the

181

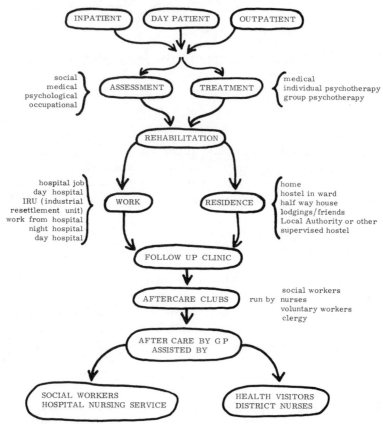

Fig. 5   Patient care and rehabilitation. Arrows represent the progress of patients. Adapted from Forrest (1973), courtesy of J W Affleck and Churchill Livingstone.

total environment of the mental hospital by introducing the concept of the **therapeutic community**.

The essence of such a community is to reproduce, in the hospital, a social life as similar as possible to life outside hospital.

The authority structure was made more democratic and an **open door** policy introduced, without, in the main, any locked wards.

An environment of permissiveness, constructive optimism, and mutual self help was encouraged.

The structure of the therapeutic community is such that authority is shared between doctors, nurses and social workers, and as far as possible, patients are given increased responsibility.

Regular communal administrative and therapeutic group meetings are held, communication generally between patient and staff is encouraged, and the priority in therapy is on rehabilitation and retraining with the development of new social and occupational skills. Work situations are used to help patients regain social insight.

The differences between treatment and rehabilitation were seen to be artificial. Treatment usually refers to more acute medical management, e.g. with drugs and psychotherapy; whereas rehabilitation implies longer term measures such as the readjustment of the acute psychotic or neurotic patient into the community, and the provision of suitable employment and rehabilitative social retraining of the chronic patient for work or just 'living' in a community or hostel. The latter group was generally made up of chronic schizophrenics, high grade subnormals and ESN individuals, inadequate personalities, and patients with recovering organic states.

Occupational therapy is an important part of this hospital therapeutic programme with occupational therapists working in close liaison with nurses, social workers and doctors. They aim to provide a skilled programme of daily activities for every patient in the hospital based on knowledge of the patient's personality, background habits, psychological problems and diagnosis. The information is acquired by personal contact and during team meetings.

Individuals are specifically helped with their psychological problems by the assessment of their response to work, and by breaking down the components of a task. Depressives, tense anxious psychoneurotics, hypomanic and schizophrenic patients are allocated tasks designed to channel their aggression creatively, to reduce excitement, encourage self-confidence, stimulate apathy into imaginative interest and to distract the psychotic from his delusions.

A wide variety of therapy is provided based on domestic life, games and vocational training. Psychodrama and music therapy are also used.

Patients are assessed by their performance in simple tasks, manual or intellectual, in regard to their initiative, concentration, memory, aptitudes, social attitudes and relationships, and suitability for return to work.

They are offered an opportunity to improve their old skills, acquire new ones, and reduce social isolation.

Occupational therapists also take part in providing group

psychotherapy and structured social retraining schemes.

The next stage in the rehabilitation programme after these measures involves attendance at an **industrial therapy unit** (ITU). Here, patients are further assessed by a disablement resettlement officer (DRO) who keeps a register of all disabled persons in the community.

The patients' aptitudes are related to simple commercial tasks and the work provided is subcontracted out from industrial firms. The patient is paid according to his productivity. Some patients never cope with more than a simple diversionary task. Others are able to manage more complicated work and are eventually referred to an **industrial resettlement unit** (IRU) where they are specifically prepared for work in the community in full employment, in a sheltered workshop, or an industrial unit staffed primarily by chronic hospital inpatients who remain there, on a semi-permanent basis, whilst continuing to live in the hospital.

The aim is to encourage patients to live and work in the community.

The further network of support arrangements for the patient in the community are organized by social workers working in conjunction with the DRO.

The further management of patients after discharge from hospital concerns the **concept of community care**.

Community care involves a community mental health service which provides comprehensive care and treatment for a defined population. This includes full hospital facilities, ideally an acute unit attached to a District General Hospital in the community and a 'back up' hospital for the care of intermediate and chronic patients.

The most efficient population size for a community service is between 150 000–200 000 – large enough to contain the basic services required and small enough to avoid anonymity of key professional workers.

Because the demand for service is potentially infinite, priorities must be decided on for the resources available within the service.

In the course of a severe psychiatric illness, a patient is likely to spend more time outside hospital than inside. Therefore, the frequency and duration of hospitalization will depend on the efficiency of the support services in the community.

It is clearly wrong to think of patients as being necessarily 'ill' when they are in hospital and 'well' when they are at home.

Thus, the community based services should be the central focus of influence with the hospital service playing a smaller part in the total management of patients.

Several **important objectives in treatment** need to be mentioned.

Firstly, there must be continuity of care, viz, the hospital doctor and his team should continue to care for the patient in the community, through out-patient attendance, discussions with the GP if the patient is at home, or with social workers – some of whom have joint appointments in both hospital and community.

The available services are integrated in many other ways, e.g. hospital patients may attend social clubs in the community, for occupational and social therapy. Hospital medical staff should take part in casework discussions with social workers and community nurses, and take part in their training. General practitioners are also involved in the community health teams.

Unfortunately, financial stringencies and inefficient organization in most areas in the UK means that in general, rehabilitation facilities for the clinically disabled are sadly lacking, and sheltered accommodation, group homes and supervised lodgings hardly available. Services for psychogeriatric patients and the young are particularly deficient.

Local authority social services were radically reorganized in 1970 following the Seebohm Report (1968). A director of Social Services was appointed in each new area. His responsibilities include:

(a) The organization and management of welfare services for the elderly, children, the homeless, the disabled and the mentally handicapped.
(b) The development of home help services.
(c) The provision of social work services in both community and hospital.
(d) Day nurseries and child guidance centres.

The probation service, however, continues to remain outside the local authorities sphere of control.

The social services department is organized on an area basis sometimes corresponding to hospital catchment areas with area and district teams of **generic social workers** who are community based and family orientated. Specialization has been abolished and social workers are trained to deal with all types of problems. Psychiatrists must, therefore, be aware of their limitations in the management of particular patients.

Social workers assist in the signing of treatment orders for patients, and are concerned with assessing and helping the social and emotional problems of the individual and the family in relation to mental illness. Their help is invaluable in the management of individuals and families with complicated emotional and social crisis that become protracted in time and wasteful of psychiatric time.

They are also called upon to deal with specific environmental problems and the organization of the often complicated strands of social help available. For example, finding accommodation for the mentally ill, taking children into care, arranging home help, negotiating the cooperation of the DRO and interviewing the families of the mentally ill.

Acute psychiatric units attached to a District General Hospital have been encouraged. Beds are allocated according to the catchment area rather than statistical norms. They serve as the nucleus for psychiatric care in the catchment area, and are staffed by doctors who may also have appointments in the catchment mental hospital which in the absence of adequate hostels, etc., is used for 'back up' facilities – viz. the placement of intermediate and long stay patients.

The Department of Health has stated that it aims at a minimum of 0.5 beds per 1000 population and 0.65 per 1000 day hospital places.

Day hospital attendance is determined by psychiatric needs, diagnostic and social circumstances. Patients may attend on a daily basis, several days per week, or at night.

A full range of treatment is provided including drugs, ECT, individual and group psychotherapy, occupational therapy and ITU. Most patients are admittable, other than the severely dis turbed, violent, or drug addicts.

An efficient, well staffed day hospital should be able to prevent 30% or more of hospital admissions and is usable as a **halfway house** after discharge from hospital.

Ideally, a **psychogeriatric day hospital** with a small **assessment unit** should also be provided.

These services are complemented by:

(a)   A hospital outpatient department service with a service for adolescents and children.

(b) Domiciliary home visits by consultant psychiatrists.

(c) A **'walk in' acute crisis intervention unit** – this may be staffed by a psychiatrist and social worker in the DGH or psychiatric unit attached to it.

Local authority day centres and social clubs provide for patients who are integrated enough to live at home but require a degree of supervision during the day. They provide recreational and vocational facilities and are staffed by social workers or a psychiatrically trained nurse.

A sheltered workshop and industrial therapy unit for psychiatric patients and the mentally handicapped are two further necessary requirements for a complete service.

Hostel accommodation is of primary importance in patient community aftercare. They are most often managed by the local authority and there are three varieties:

1 Hostels or 'group homes' for the homeless cater for individuals who have spent a long time in hospital cut off from their families; or people who require 'shelter' rather than being a medical or social responsibility. The aim of this type of hostel or home is to help people 'stand on their feet' again and achieve some degree of personal and social independence with a minimum of supervision, or no supervision at all.

2 Hostels for patients requiring a degree of supervision and support from staff with some psychiatric training, e.g. those taking psychotropic drugs, chronic schizophrenics, subnormals and epileptics.

3 'Hospital hostels' for the longstay emotionally disturbed patient. Highly qualified personnel are required with support and guidance from psychiatrists and social workers. They should be sited near the acute unit.

All professional staff involved in the care of the mentally ill should liaise closely with **voluntary agencies**, e.g. The Richmond Fellowship, who provide supervised hostel accommodation, the AA (Alcoholics Anonymous), Narcotics Anonymous and marriage guidance clinics.

Meetings between their staff and professional workers in the community should be arranged for the periodic discussion of problems, the planning of strategy and the assessment of future needs.

The combination of new attitudes towards mental hospital patients the therapeutic community approach, advances in psycho-pharmacology, active rehabilitation and community care, have resulted in a significant drop in the numbers of chronic mental hospital patients, as well as acute admissions.

Many mental hospitals are 'running down' their numbers and the residual population is now composed of patients with dementia rather than schizophrenia.

'Institutional neurosis' (doctor, nurse and patient apathy, lack of concern and low morale, and loss of personal identity and emotional withdrawal of patients) has almost disappeared.

Despite the progress outlined, many patients are discharged into the community without adequate provision for their aftercare. They lose contact with the social services, wander from area to area and exist in conditions of extreme emotional, material and social deprivation.

The current vogue for discharging patients into the community may be reaching saturation point.

Thus it is clear that mental hospitals are not necessarily redundant, and that there are many patients who cannot cope outside a mental hospital setting, especially in view of the fact that the community care ideal is far from being realized.

The hospital services deal with only a fraction of psychiatrically ill patients.

General practitioner surveys indicate that 1/5–1/10 of the total population is or will be mentally disturbed at any one time and that the majority are either treated in the context of the community or remain untreated.

In the final analysis, **it is the general practitioner** who is the first link in the treatment chain of psychiatric patients. Inevitably, they occupy a large part of his time. Ultimately, GPs should receive enough basic training in the management of psychiatric patients to be able to undertake a limited amount of psychotherapy and drug treatment. Their close relationship to the family, and intimate knowledge of the domestic problems and the patient's background, gives them a unique advantage in treatment.

Generally, the effectiveness, quality and quantity of psychiatric work undertaken by a GP varies according to his interest, aptitude for psychotherapy and training. He should ideally be able to cope with many of his chronic patients, addicts, emotionally disturbed and inadequate individuals without recourse to the mental health services.

22 More Advanced Reading

1 General comprehensive textbooks

Forrest, A. (Ed.) (1973), *Companion to psychiatric studies* Vols. 1 & 2. Edinburgh: Churchill Livingstone.

Freedman, A. M., Kaplan, H. I. & Sadock, B. J. (1972), *Modern synopsis of comprehensive textbook of psychiatry.* Baltimore: Williams & Wilkins.

Sim, M. (1974), *Guide to psychiatry* (3rd Ed.). Edinburgh: Churchill Livingstone.

Slater, E. & Roth, M. (1969), In *Clinical psychiatry* (3rd Ed.), Mayer-Gross, Slater, & Roth. London: Bailliere Tindall & Cassell.

2 More specialized topics

Aldrich, C. K. (1966), *An introduction to dynamic psychiatry.* London: McGraw Hill.

Altschul, A. (1973), *Psychiatric nursing* (4th Ed.). Nurses' Aids Series. London: Bailliere Tindall & Cassell.

Berne, E. (1968), *Games people play.* London: Penguin.

Burr, J. (1970), *Nursing the psychiatric patient* (2nd Ed.). London: Bailliere Tindall & Cassell.

Clarke, A. D. B. & Clarke, A. M. (1975), *Recent advances in the study of subnormality* (Revised Ed.). MIND monograph.

Department of Health and Social Security (1971), *Hospital services for the mentally ill.* London: HMSO.

Department of Health and Social Security (1973), *Services for mental illness related to old age.* London: HMSO.

Feighner, J. B., Robins, E., Guze, S. B., Woodcraft, R. A., Winokur, G. & Miroz, R. (1972), Diagnostic criteria for use in psychiatric research. *Arch. gen. Psychiat.,* **26,** 57–63.

Fleming, A. C. & Paterson, H. F. (1969), *Mental disorder and the law.* Edinburgh: Churchill Livingstone.

190

Freud, S. (1962), *Two short accounts of psycho-analysis.* London: Penguin.

Granville-Grossman, K. (Ed.) (1976), *Recent advances in clinical psychiatry*, Vol. 2. Edinburgh: Churchill Livingstone. (See also Vol. 1, 1971.)

Masters: W. H. & Johnson, V. E. (1966), *Human sexual response.* London: Churchill Livingstone.

Masters, W. H. & Johnson, V. E. (1970), *Human sexual inadequacy.* London: Churchill Livingstone.

Priest, R. G. (1972), The impact of the abortion act: a psychiatrist's observations. *Brit. J. Psychiat.*, **121**, 293–297.

Priest, R. G. (1973), A new approach to sleep disorders. *Gazetta Sanitaria*, **22**, 1–12.

Priest, R. G. (1975), Discussion of papers by Merskey, Buhrich and Gadd. 1. Hysteria. *Br. J. Med. Psychol.*, **48**, 371–373.

Priest, R. G. (1976), The homeless person and the psychiatric services: an Edinburgh survey. *Brit. J. Psychiat.*, **128**, 128–136.

Priest, R. G. (1977), Recognition of the suicidal patient. *J. Int. Med. Res.*, **5**, Supplement 1, 157–163.

Priest, R. G. (1977), Choice of antidepressants. *The Practitioner*, Special number 'Choice of Treatment', 487–900.

Priest, R. G. (1977), Sadness, hate and suicide. *Proc. Ciba Symposium on Depression, Malta*, 1976. Horsham, England: Ciba Laboratories.

Priest, R. G. (1978), Psychiatric indications for termination of pregnancy. In *Current themes in psychiatry*, Gaind, R. (Ed.). London: Macmillan.

Priest, R. G. (1978), Sleep and its disorders. In *Current themes in psychiatry*, Gaind, R. (Ed.). London: Macmillan.

Priest, R. G. & Steinert, J. (1977), *Insanity: the major psychiatric disorders.* London: Macdonald and Evans.

Ratoff, L., Cooper, B. & Rockett, D. (1973), Seebohm and the NHS survey of medico-social liaison. *British Medical Journal*, **2**, 51–53.

Sahakian, W. S. (Ed.) (1969), *Psychotherapy and counselling: studies in technique.* Chicago: Rand McNally.

Sargent, W. & Slater, E. (1963), *An introduction to physical methods of treatment in psychiatry.* Edinburgh: Livingstone.

Tooley, R. H. (1967), *Mental Health Act 1959: a review.* London: Medical Protection Society.

3   For reference only

Dunham, H. W. (1965), *Community and schizophrenia*. Detroit: Wayne State University.

Faris, R. E. L. & Dunham, H. W. (1960), *An ecological study of schizophrenia and other psychoses*. New York: Hafner Publishing Co.

Goldberg, E. M. & Morrison, S. L. (1963), Schizophrenia and social class. *Brit. J. Psychiat.*, **109,** 785–802.

Hare, E. H. (1956), Family setting and the urban distribution of schizophrenia. *J. ment. Sci.*, **102,** 753–760.

Hare, E. H. (1956), Mental illness and social conditions in Bristol. *J. ment. Sci.*, **102,** 349–357.

Rosen, I. (Ed.) (1964), *Pathology and treatment of sexual deviations*. London: Oxford University Press.

Rutter, M. & Hersov, L. (1977), *Child psychiatry*. Oxford: Blackwell Scientific Publications.

Wyeth Laboratories (undated), *Compulsory hospital admission and a glossary of mental disorders*. Taplow: Wyeth Laboratories.

Appendix I

Name and address memory test

Tell the patient:
'I would like to test your memory. I am going to read out an imaginary name and address. Please say each line back to me after I read it.'

'Mr A. B. Carter'	(wait for reply)
'98 Grange Road'	(wait for reply)
'West Ham'	(wait for reply)

If the patient makes an error during the administration, he is told the correct response at once, and he is asked to repeat that line again. The administration then continues. At the end of the administration, ask: 'Now can you repeat the whole name and address?' and his answer is recorded. (If there is no answer at first, prompt with 'Mr ?'.)

The procedure should be repeated once (if there are no errors) or twice (if errors were made in immediate recall) to ensure good registration. Each repetition is introduced briefly by: 'Let's do that again now' or 'Shall we do that one more time?'. After the final administration, a note is made of the time at that point.

For an interval of somewhere between 5 and 20 minutes, the patient is distracted by talking to him about other matters, or doing other tests, then a note is made of the time once more and he is asked: 'Can you remember that imaginary name and address I gave you?'.

The answers are recorded as in the following typical case:

Test address	1st recall	2nd recall	3rd recall	Delayed recall
Mr A. B. Carter	Carter	Carter	A. B. Carter	Carter
98 Grange Road	98 –	98 West Road	98 Grange Street	98 West Street
West Ham	West Ham	West Ham	West Ham	West Ham
			Time: 10.37 a.m.	Time: 10.48 a.m.

Notes

1 The advantage of this test is its relative simplicity and the fact that no special test materials are required (other than pencil and paper).

2 Although extreme results (e.g. no recall at all after ten minutes, or completely perfect recall) may be of value, intermediate results are often difficult to interpret. The value of this test is that it can be repeated (using the same time interval as before) to see whether the patient's mental state is improving or deteriorating.

3 If you wish to do the test again, it is in order to invent another address of similar complexity, e.g.:

Mr B. C. Davies

45 Green Lane

East Croydon

4 The instructions have been spelled out in detail so that this can be used as a **standardized** test – that is, there should be as little variation as possible in the way that different people use it.

Index

195